Group
Techniques

Group Techniques

THIRD EDITION

Gerald Corey
California State University, Fullerton

Marianne Schneider Corey
Private Practice

Patrick Callanan
Private Practice

J. Michael Russell
California State University, Fullerton

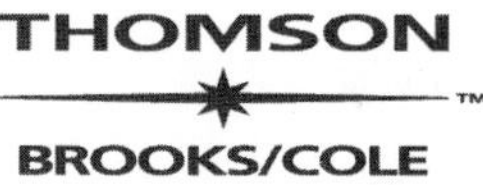

Australia • Canada • Mexico • Singapore • Spain • United Kingdom • United States

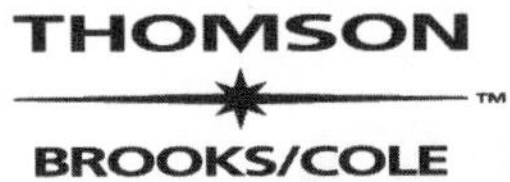

Sponsoring Editor: *Julie Martinez*
Marketing Manager: *Caroline Concilla*
Marketing Assistant: *Mary Ho*
Assistant Editor: *Shelley Gesicki*
Editorial Assistant: *Amy Lam*
Project Editor: *Kim Svetich-Will*
Production Service: *The Cooper Company*
Manuscript Editor: *Kay Mikel*
Permissions Editor: *Sue Ewing*
Cover Design: *Andy Norris*
Cover Photo: *Adalberto Rios Szalay/Sexto Sol*
Interior Design: *Vernon Boes*
Print Buyer: *Kristine Waller*
Compositor: *Scratchgravel Publishing Services*
Printing and Binding: *Webcom Ltd.*

Printed in Canada

3 4 5 6 7 06 05

Library of Congress Control Number: 2002113771

ISBN 0-534-61267-9

Brooks/Cole–Thomson Learning
511 Forest Lodge Road
Pacific Grove, CA 93950
USA

Asia
Thomson Learning
5 Shenton Way #01-01
UIC Building
Singapore 068808

Australia/New Zealand
Thomson Learning
102 Dodds Street
Southbank, Victoria 3006
Australia

Canada
Nelson
1120 Birchmount Road
Toronto, Ontario M1K 5G4
Canada

Europe/Middle East/Africa
Thomson Learning
High Holborn House
50/51 Bedford Row
London WC1R 4LR
United Kingdom

Latin America
Thomson Learning
Seneca, 53
Colonia Polanco
11560 Mexico D.F.
Mexico

Spain/Portugal
Paraninfo
Calle Magallanes, 25
28015 Madrid
Spain

Our book is dedicated to
the people who have been members in our groups,
especially those in our residential workshops,
who gave us the opportunity to learn more.

ABOUT THE AUTHORS

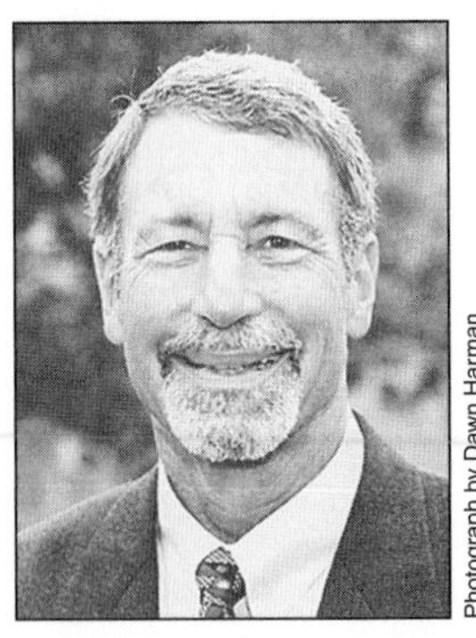
Photograph by Dawn Harman

GERALD COREY is Professor Emeritus of Human Services at California State University, Fullerton. He received his doctorate in counseling from the University of Southern California. He is a Diplomate in Counseling Psychology, American Board of Professional Psychology; a licensed psychologist; a National Certified Counselor; a Fellow of the American Psychological Association (Counseling Psychology); and a Fellow of the Association for Specialists in Group Work.

Jerry received the Outstanding Professor of the Year Award from California State University, Fullerton in 1991 and was the recipient of the Association for Specialists in Group Work Eminent Career Award in 2001. He teaches both undergraduate and graduate courses in group counseling, as well as courses in experiential groups, the theory and practice of counseling, and ethics in counseling practice. With his colleagues he has conducted workshops in the United States, Germany, Ireland, Belgium, Scotland, Mexico, and China, with a special focus on training in group counseling. He often presents workshops for professional organizations, special intensive courses at various universities, and residential training and supervision workshops for group leaders. In his leisure time, Jerry likes to travel, hike and bicycle in the mountains, and drive his 1931 Model A Ford.

Recent publications by Jerry Corey, all with Brooks/Cole, include:

Theory and Practice of Group Counseling, Sixth Edition (and *Student Manual*) (2004)
Clinical Supervision in the Helping Professions: A Practical Guide (2003, with Robert Haynes and Patrice Moulton)
Issues and Ethics in the Helping Professions, Sixth Edition (2003, with Marianne Schneider Corey and Patrick Callanan)
Becoming a Helper, Fourth Edition (2003, with Marianne Schneider Corey)
Groups: Process and Practice, Sixth Edition (2002, with Marianne Schneider Corey)
I Never Knew I Had a Choice, Seventh Edition (2002, with Marianne Schneider Corey)
Theory and Practice of Counseling and Psychotherapy, Sixth Edition (and *Student Manual*) (2001)
Case Approach to Counseling and Psychotherapy, Fifth Edition (2001)
The Art of Integrative Counseling (2001)

Jerry is co-author, with his daughters Cindy Corey and Heidi Jo Corey, of an orientation-to-college book entitled *Living and Learning* (1997), published by Wadsworth. He is also co-author (with Barbara Herlihy) of *Boundary Issues in Counseling: Multiple Roles and Responsibilities* (1997) and *ACA Ethical Standards Casebook*, Fifth Edition (1996), both published by the American Counseling Association.

He has also made three videos on various aspects of counseling practice:

Student Video and Workbook for the Art of Integrative Counseling (2001, with Robert Haynes)
The Evolution of a Group: Student Video and Workbook (2000, with Marianne Schneider Corey and Robert Haynes)
Ethics in Action: CD-ROM (2003, with Marianne Schneider Corey and Robert Haynes)

All of these student videos and workbooks (and CD-ROM) are available through Brooks/Cole–Thomson Learning.

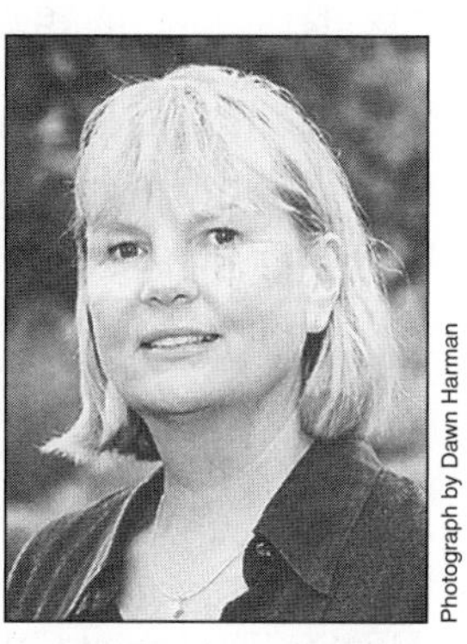
Photograph by Dawn Harman

MARIANNE SCHNEIDER COREY is a licensed marriage and family therapist in California and is a National Certified Counselor. She received her master's degree in marriage, family, and child counseling from Chapman College. She is a Fellow of the Association for Specialists in Group Work and was the recipient of this organization's Eminent Career Award in 2001. She also holds memberships in the American Counseling Association; the Association for Spiritual, Ethical, and Religious Values in Counseling; the Association for Counselor Education and Supervision (both national and regional); the Western Psychological Association; and the Association for Specialists in Group Work.

Marianne has been actively involved in leading groups for different populations, providing training and supervision workshops in group process, facilitating a self-exploration group for graduate students in counseling, and co-facilitating training groups for group counselors and weeklong residential workshops in personal growth. She sees groups as the most effective format in which to work with clients and finds it the most rewarding for her personally. With her husband, Jerry, Marianne has conducted training workshops, continuing education seminars, and personal growth groups in Germany, Ireland, Belgium, Mexico, and China, as well as regularly doing these workshops in the United States. In her free time, Marianne enjoys traveling, reading, visiting with friends, and hiking.

Marianne has co-authored several articles in group work, as well as the following books with Brooks/Cole:

Issues and Ethics in the Helping Professions, Sixth Edition (2003, with Gerald Corey and Patrick Callanan)
Becoming a Helper, Fourth Edition (2003, with Gerald Corey)
Groups: Process and Practice, Sixth Edition (2002, with Gerald Corey)
I Never Knew I Had a Choice, Seventh Edition (2002, with Gerald Corey)

Marianne has made several videos (with accompanying student workbooks) for Brooks/Cole–Thomson Learning: *Ethics in Action*: CD-ROM; *Ethics in Action* (Institutional Version); and *The Evolution of a Group*. This last video, *The Evolution of a Group,* is very appropriate for use as a companion to *Group Techniques* since it illustrates the unfolding of each of the stages of a group and highlights techniques aimed at deepening group interaction and member self-exploration.

Marianne and Jerry have been married since 1964. They have two adult daughters, Heidi and Cindy. Marianne grew up in Germany and has kept in close contact with her family there.

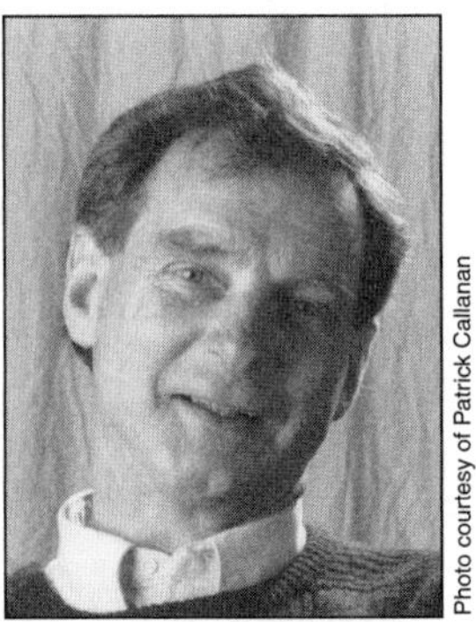

PATRICK CALLANAN is a licensed marriage and family therapist in private practice in Santa Ana, California. In 1973 he graduated with a bachelor's degree in Human Services from California State University at Fullerton, and then received his master's degree in professional psychology from United States International University in 1976. In his private practice he works with individuals, couples, families, and groups.

Patrick is on the part-time faculty of the Human Services Program at California State University, Fullerton, where he regularly teaches an internship course. He also offers his time each year to the university to assist in training and supervising group leaders and coteaches an undergraduate course in ethical and professional issues. Along with Marianne Schneider Corey and Gerald Corey, he received an Award for Contributions to the Field of Professional Ethics by the Association for Spiritual, Ethical, and Religious Values in Counseling in 1986.

Patrick has also co-authored, with Marianne and Gerald Corey, the following book (published by Brooks/Cole): *Issues and Ethics in the Helping Professions,* Sixth Edition (2003). In his free time, Patrick enjoys reading, walking fast, and playing golf.

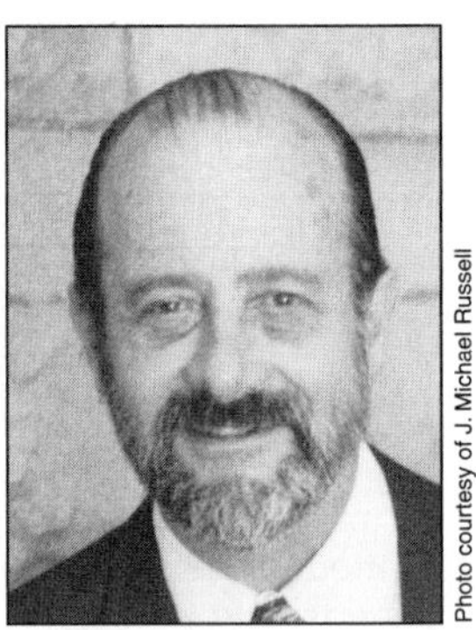

J. MICHAEL RUSSELL is Professor of Philosophy and Human Services at California State University at Fullerton, a psychoanalyst in private practice, and a core faculty member and training analyst of the Newport Psychoanalytic Institute. He has been leading workshops and teaching courses in personal growth since 1971, when he obtained his doctorate in philosophy from the University of California at Santa Barbara. His philosophical interest in self-deception broadened into courses he teaches in philosophical assumptions of psychotherapy, existentialism, death and meaning, theories and techniques of counseling, case analysis, and group leadership, and into workshops he conducts in leadership training. He became a National Certified Counselor in 1984, a registered Research Psychoanalyst in 1985, and a Graduate Psychoanalyst in 1988. He is a member of several professional organizations, including the American Counseling Association, the Association for Specialists in Group Work, the American Philosophical Association, and the American Philosophical Practitioners Association. Some biography, course materials, and articles are available on his Web page: http://jmichaelrussell.org. His publications include the following:

"Philosophical Counseling Is Not a Distinct Field: Reflections of a Philosophical Practitioner." *International Journal of Philosophical Practice,* Vol. 1, No. 1, Summer 2001.

"The In-Reach–Outreach Project of the Human Services Department at CSU Fullerton" (with Kanel, Russell, Hogan-Garcia, Kim-Goh, and Corey). *Human Services Education,* Fall 2001.

"What Are Philosophers Good For?" *The Philosophers' Magazine,* Summer 1998.

"Perversion, Eating Disorders, and Sex Roles." *International Forum for Psychoanalysis,* 1992, 1, 98–103.

"The Human Services Program at California State University, Fullerton" (with Corey, Corey, Ramirez, and Wright). *Journal of Counseling and Human Services,* May 1986.
"Desires Don't Cause Actions," *Journal of Mind and Behavior,* Winter 1984.
"Ethical Considerations in Using Group Techniques" (with Corey, Corey, and Callanan). *Journal for Specialists in Group Work,* September 1982.
"Reflection and Self-Deception." *Journal for Research in Phenomenology, 1981,* Volume II.
"A Report of a Weeklong Residential Workshop for Personal Growth" (with Corey, Corey, and Callanan). *Journal for Specialists in Group Work,* November 1980.
"How to Think About Thinking: A Preliminary Map." *Journal of Mind and Behavior,* 1980, 1(1), 45–62.
"Sartre's Theory of Sexuality." *Journal of Humanistic Psychology,* 1979, 19(2), 35–45.
"Sartre, Therapy, and Expanding the Concept of Responsibility." *American Journal of Psychoanalysis,* 1978, 38(3), 259–269.
"Saying, Feeling, and Self-Deception." *Behaviorism,* 1978, 6(1), 27–43.
"Psychotherapy and Quasi-Performantive Speech," *Behaviorism,* 1973, 1(2), 77–86.

CONTENTS

PREFACE

Since the four of us began working together in 1972, we have been involved in almost every aspect of group work as members, leaders, teachers, and workshop conductors. In the course of this long association, we have found ourselves continually faced with questions about techniques in groups—their place, their usefulness, their abuse. In many of our training workshops we have observed beginning leaders having difficulty using techniques appropriately and effectively.

Our primary assumption in this book is that techniques are never the main course in group work. This assumption has many implications. It puts the focus on the members and the leader and on the quality of the interactions between them. Techniques are means, not ends, and their primary aim is to increase knowledge and awareness on the part of the group members. Techniques are fundamentally at the service of the group members, not the group therapist.

To avoid having the techniques described in this book used as the primary focus of group work, we concentrate on showing leaders how to develop and use techniques in their own evolving groups. You can best use this book by reading a chapter, putting the book down, and then asking yourself what relevance the techniques described have for you in your situation and how they might be applied. We hope you will not borrow our techniques verbatim and use them without consideration for the members of your groups and their unique relationships with you and with one another.

In addition to being direct responses to problems presented by participants in groups we have led, the techniques in this book bear the stamp of our own therapists, of leaders of groups and workshops in which we have been members, and of a great many writers with various theoretical orientations. These techniques did not arise in a vacuum, and we provide a selected bibliography at the end of the book to further your thinking about how you might develop your therapeutic style as a group counselor.

We expect that this book will stimulate your interest in the broad field of working with people in groups and in the philosophical and ethical dimensions of what you do. Such an interest could lead you to think about theories of therapy, to further your own therapy, to engage in exchanges of ideas rather than being professionally isolated, and to participate in professional workshops. It could also lead you to an interest in supervision, whether in the formal sense of learning or in the informal sense of working with respected colleagues.

In this third edition, we have given more attention to explaining the therapeutic rationale for the various techniques we describe. At times we link particular techniques to a theoretical orientation to group counseling described in detail in Corey (2004) *Theory and Practice of Group Counseling,* Sixth Edition. This book addresses 10 theoretical approaches to group counseling, and specific chapter references refer readers to these comprehensive discussions.

This book is for students and practitioners in any human services field, from counseling psychology to social work, where the group is an accepted modality. In the classroom it can be a valuable auxiliary text in basic group courses and in a practicum in group work. The techniques described are most appropriately used with counseling groups with an open-ended agenda. In practice the book can be used to stimulate thinking and creativity in one's approach to group work, and it can be used in conjunction with supervision. Intended readers include psychiatric nurses, social workers, counselors, psychologists, ministers, marriage and family therapists, teachers, and mental health professionals and paraprofessionals who lead groups.

In this third edition of *Group Techniques* we have fine-tuned the various techniques. Although we take an eclectic stance and avoid a single theoretical bias, we emphasize throughout that a sound theoretical rationale is an essential guide when using any technique. We hope that the tone and spirit of this book will encourage group leaders to develop their own therapeutic styles. At the same time, we recommend necessary cautions, both procedural and ethical, as group leaders design and implement various techniques.

Guide to Use of *Groups in Action: Evolution and Challenges* DVD and Workbook

Groups in Action: Evolution and Challenges consists of two different interactive programs. The first program, entitled *Evolution of a Group,* is a two-hour educational video designed to bring to life the development of a group at a three-day residential workshop co-facilitated by Marianne Schneider Corey and Gerald Corey. The group workshop included people who were group members willing to explore their own issues and concerns. They were neither actors following a script nor were they role-playing the topics. The second program, entitled *Challenges Facing Group Leaders,* is a 90-minute educational video designed to address some of the most problematic situations that group counselors often encounter. In this particular program the Coreys co-facilitated a group that was composed of members who role-played a variety of scenarios depicting critical issues in a group. The participants of the second program did not follow a script; rather they improvised around themes that typically evolve in groups. At times the participants engaged in role playing and often times this moved into real personal involvement and genuine interaction in the group. In short, the participants demonstrate a blend of both role playing and drawing upon their experiences from the present and the past, both in their roles as group members and leaders.

The first program, *Evolution of a Group,* illustrates significant group process and leadership techniques in a therapeutic group. You will see the development of the group process and how the co-leaders facilitated that process as the group moved through the four stages: initial, transition, working, and ending—which correspond to Chapters 4 to 7 of *Group Techniques.*

In the initial stage, the focus is on building trust and focusing on the here-and-now. The leaders set the stage by exploring ground rules for the group operation and assisting members in developing goals for this group. In the transition stage, identifying and challenging member fears, hesitations, and resistance are the main topics. The level of trust is deepening, and members begin reluctantly to talk about personal material. The working stage is characterized by a high level of trust, clearer goals, and members exploring feelings, ideas, and beliefs. Group cohesiveness is high, and members interact with each other with less reliance on the leaders. In the ending stage, the group members review what they have learned, discussing how they will actually put those learnings into action, and prepare for ending the group.

Throughout the DVD program you will see the Coreys co-leading and facilitating the group process from beginning to end. The co-leaders utilize a variety of group techniques from various group treatment approaches. It is the combination of viewing both the implementation of group leadership techniques and the movement of the group through the four stages of group process that makes this a unique DVD training program. This multimedia integration is aimed at expanding the learning experience for students of group counseling.

The second program, *Challenges Facing Group Leaders,* consists of improvisational enactments of problematic scenarios and critical incidents in a group. The Coreys encouraged the participants of this second program to be themselves as much as possible, even though they were at times enacting different roles. Some of the scenarios that are enacted include: working with members who do not want to be a part of the group; dealing with a group when they are making little progress; addressing conflict; dealing with silence; exploring a member's reactions to being left with unresolved feelings about a prior group session; working with members who are uncomfortable with expressing emotions; addressing a member's concern over feeling pressured to talk; managing a member who assumes a role of assistant leader; dealing with trust issues and concerns about confidentiality; working with a quiet member; and the challenges in dealing with a range of difficult behaviors in groups. A significant part of this second program involves addressing the ways that diversity influences group process. A few of the issues pertaining to diversity include: experiencing identity concerns; feeling different from others; dealing with stereotypes; speaking in one's primary language; looking to leaders for answers; and looking at the ways in which people are both the same and different.

The second program is intended to teach ways of understanding and effectively working with a range of challenging situations that group counselors frequently encounter, especially during the early stages of a group. A few of the key points that are illustrated in the *Challenges Facing Group Leaders* program are listed below:

- Group work is slow and tedious at times, which demands patience on the leader's part.
- Group facilitators have the responsibility of creating safety within a group.
- The earlier phases of a group are critical in terms of laying a solid foundation for work at the later stages.
- Work takes place at all stages of group—not only during the beginning stages. How effectively a leader deals with challenges from group members at an early stage determines how effective a group will eventually become.

As students view this DVD program and respond to the questions in the accompanying workbook, we hope they will do so with an openness to learn about how group process works—and with a willingness to examine their own beliefs as a group leader. This program can provide the experiential piece that helps students more concretely understand the nature of group process, and it can be a catalyst that prompts them into self-exploration. The art of group leadership is far more than a technical endeavor; it involves a group leader's capacity to use his or her intuition and human responses. To be sure, effective group leaders need a theoretical grasp of group process along with the knowledge and skill base to make effective interventions in a group. Competent group leaders possess self-understanding, knowledge of dynamics of behavior and group process, and technical skills in group facilitation.

Acknowledgments

A number of individuals have provided us with input that has enhanced the third edition of *Group Techniques.* We are indebted to the following people who offered both a prerevision review and a review of the final manuscript: Darcy Haag Granello, The Ohio State University; Maria Saxionis, Bridgewater State College; Conni Sharp, Pittsburg State University; William Wheeler, Mississippi College; and Robert Witchel, Indiana University of Pennsylvania.

The members of the Brooks/Cole team continue to offer support for all our projects. It is a delight to work with a dedicated staff of professionals who go out of their way to give their best. These people include Julie Martinez, counseling editor; Cat Broz, who coordinated the reviewing process; Kim Svetich-Will, the production manager for the project; and Cecile Joyner and Benjamin Kolstad of The Cooper Company, the production editors. We want to give special recognition and appreciation to Kay Mikel, the manuscript editor of this edition, whose superb editorial skills kept this book reader friendly. Thanks go to Mimi Lawson for her work in compiling the index.

Gerald Corey
Marianne Schneider Corey
Patrick Callanan
Michael Russell

CHAPTER ONE

The Role of Techniques

Introduction

The title of this book is *Group Techniques,* but what exactly is a counseling "technique"? This word is not as simple to define as you might think. Virtually anything a group leader does could be viewed as a technique, including being silent, suggesting a new behavior, inviting a client to explore a conflict, maintaining eye contact, arranging seating, offering reactions to members, and presenting interpretations.

We generally use the term *technique* in a more precise way to refer to a leader's explicit and direct request of a member to focus on material, augment or exaggerate affect, practice behavior, or solidify insight. This definition includes the following procedures: conducting the initial interview, in which a prospective member is asked to focus on his or her reasons for wanting to join a group; asking a nonproductive group to clarify the direction it wants to take; asking a member to role-play a specific situation; asking a member to practice a behavior; encouraging a member to repeat certain words or to complete a sentence; helping a member summarize what she or he has learned from a group session; challenging a member's beliefs; and working with the cognitions that influence a member's behavior. We also consider as techniques those procedures aimed at helping group leaders get a sense of the direction the group might want to pursue.

When we facilitate a group, we use a variety of techniques that flow from many theoretical approaches. We adapt the techniques to fit the needs of the group participants rather than attempting to fit the members to our techniques. When implementing techniques, we consider members' readiness to confront their problems, their cultural background, their value system, their trust in us as leaders, and the stage in the development of the group.

Avoiding the Misuse of Techniques

Misconceptions about the use of techniques abound. When we give workshops on groups, participants sometimes ask us to suggest techniques for working with specific clients. The implication seems to be that there is a "proper technique" for every situation. Perhaps for some models of group counseling, such as behavior modification, specific methods are appropriate to achieve well-defined behavioral outcomes. In many types of groups, however, the techniques that are most useful grow out of the work of the participants and are tailored to the situations that evolve in a particular session.

Given our assumption that techniques are means and not ends, we naturally have some concerns about how this book will be used:

- Will the book contribute to the problem of group leaders' overemphasizing techniques?
- Will readers memorize specific devices and use them thoughtlessly rather than treating them as a means to deepen their own therapeutic inventiveness and judgment?

In both cases, of course, we hope not. Instead, we want you to use your own creativity and learn to develop techniques spontaneously from the work being done.

It is impossible to predict what the exact nature of a group will be. Relying on a recipe-book approach to therapeutic techniques may provide opportunities to try different procedures, but surely it does not replace the main function of a group leader. An excellent cook creates a different dish each time, and we encourage you to approach your groups with a little of the same creativity. Use your intuition, use what is available at the moment, and trust your own sensitivity and judgment.

Paying attention to the obvious. Techniques can deepen feelings that are already present, and they should preferably grow out of what is already taking place. When a person says, "I'm feeling lonely," for example, it is appropriate to introduce a technique addressing loneliness to help move this feeling further. For this reason, we generally prefer to include the members in the selection of group themes rather than to select a theme arbitrarily. This is not a hard-and-fast rule; many group practitioners work effectively with preselected techniques, exercises, and themes. Indeed, for certain populations, this approach is indicated. Many short-term structured groups make use of topics and exercises to help members learn. Thus, techniques are employed to help members accomplish their personal goals within the framework of the group's basic purpose.

In the groups we lead, we tend to use techniques to initiate material at the beginning of a group and often also to summarize material at the end. We also use techniques for elaborating on what is already happening, letting members lead the way. We find that it is best to follow the energy and the clues provided by the members rather than being overly directive.

Most groups have moments of stagnation or resistance. It is easy in these situations but often unwise to employ a technique to get things moving quickly rather than paying attention to the important material being presented, mainly the resistance. It can be therapeutically useful to teach group members how to assess what is occurring in the group process and how to mobilize the group's energy. By looking around the room, for example, you may notice that members show signs of being disengaged; they appear to be bored, they are fidgeting, or they are frustrated. We think the best technique at such times is to ask the members about their sense of what's happening. You might say: "I'm willing to work hard to help you get what you came for. I'm also aware that many of you do not seem interested. Few of you are speaking up, there is a good deal of fidgeting, and people are not responding to one another. I'd like to hear from each of you what is happening with you now." You can then share your reactions at the moment, or you can save them until all members have expressed what they are experiencing. Avoid trying technique after technique to stimulate movement in a situation such as this. Deal with what is actually occurring within the group by describing without judgment the behavior you are observing and by encouraging the members to decide what they want to do about their level of involvement in the group.

In addition, when considering whether to introduce a technique, take into account the stage of the group's development. For instance, you can expect trust to be an issue at the initial stage of a group. A group may be somewhat silent and cautious at this point in its existence. To introduce a technique to get things moving is to ignore the obvious and to impose a dynamic that is either premature for the group or that forces a process. Doing so tends to interfere with the group's natural development. By introducing a technique that stresses and clarifies what is happening, you augment the process rather than interfere with it.

Maintaining flexibility. As leaders of groups, we encourage you to develop flexibility about which material to work with; it is important that you be ready to go wherever the members may want to go. Thus, be prepared to abandon a technique that seems to lead nowhere or to modify it as needed. We once witnessed a therapist demonstrating work with an angry woman. He kept urging her to hit a pillow with her hands, apparently failing to notice that she was already twisting the pillow. A more insightful approach might have been to work with what twisting the pillow meant to her. To take a different illustration, a leader may determine that a client needs to pursue an issue with her father. The leader may introduce a technique designed to accentuate her sadness and yet should be alert to whether or not she is actually feeling sad.

In a group therapy session we supervised, a violent patient kept reiterating that he was "different." The leader tried to focus the client on dealing with his violent feelings rather than exploring his more pressing concern about being different. Either theme could have been worked with, but the outcome might have been more useful to the client had the leader gone with the client's feeling of being different. By being open to members' needs at the moment, the group leader can assess what techniques can be most effective.

When material is presented by a member, the direction you choose to follow and the techniques you will use depend to a great extent on who you are as a person and your theoretical orientation. If you were to observe 10 different therapists working with the same material brought up by a client, each of the therapists could be working quite differently, yet each one could be helpful in a variety of ways.

Although it is possible to make mistakes because of insensitivity to promising and pressing material, don't become too anxious about pursuing the "right" or the "most pressing" material. There is often no single "right" way to proceed. If you become too focused on doing exactly the right thing at the right time, you are likely to stifle your creativity and miss important clues provided by group members.

Often, several directions are equally worth pursuing. When we are asked why we chose one direction rather than another in a given situation, we frequently believe we could also have taken the work in a different direction. Besides our theoretical orientation and therapeutic style, our own interests and level of energy come into play. Techniques are seldom picked randomly; rather, they are connected to a therapeutic purpose.

The Therapeutic Relationship

Much of the opportunity for significant change is based on the members' relationship with the group leader. Just as many of the behaviors we label maladaptive had their origins in faulty early relationships, new and more appropriate behaviors can be cemented through the new relationship with the leader and group members. If this relationship is inauthentic, superficial, or otherwise impoverished, we doubt that clients will make significant strides in making changes. Changes must be tried out, and the therapeutic relationship provides this testing ground. Let's look at two issues in the use of techniques that illustrate the significance of the therapeutic relationship: timing and avoiding self-deception.

Timing the use of techniques. A critical skill in group work is using techniques with consideration for whether clients are prepared for change. When we push beyond clients' readiness to change, we violate their integrity. To assault defenses without consideration for their importance in maintaining equilibrium is to expose clients to possible psychological damage. No technique will provide you with information on how ready clients are to give up their defenses. You need intelligence, wisdom, and, above all, a concerned attentiveness to your relationship with your clients. This relationship provides them and you with the hold on reality clients need to move away from nonproductive and excessively defensive conduct.

As group members learn to trust you, they are likely to move toward change. In the absence of such a relationship, they are being asked to trust techniques without any sense of what the leader is all about. Clients in that position do well to resist. The therapist who pays attention to the leader/client relationship develops a sixth sense that makes it possible to gauge the course of therapy and to judge the optimum time for gently pushing clients into areas previously feared. This skill is above and beyond technique. To some degree it is a part of the therapist's makeup, but it can be refined through training and supervision.

Avoiding self-deception in using techniques. Techniques can be powerful sources for emotional release and can generate tremendous energy in the therapeutic group. But they can easily mask the relationship between the leader and the members. When the storm has subsided, any insights gained can be easily dismissed by clients as having been brought about by something foreign to their own resources: the power of a special environment or the magic of the leader's technical skills. At the other extreme, because of the impact of a cathartic moment, clients may cling to the false belief that the issue has now been worked on and is finished. Catharsis can be exciting, and yet it can feed a false sense of change. The leader who is anxious to produce a heavy emotional session may use techniques to generate such emotion without being sensitive to the need to explore the material to a deeper level and to gain some comprehension of its meaning and implications.

Choosing Techniques for Various Types of Groups

The type of group you lead will determine, to a large degree, the appropriateness of various techniques. Some techniques may be ideally suited for a therapeutic group, yet they may not be appropriate for certain groups with an educational focus. The majority of the techniques we describe in this book work best in therapeutic groups. Some of the techniques we describe in the chapters on the transition and working stages, for example, would not be suitable for a short-term structured group with children. However, our purpose is not to present techniques with the idea that you will copy them. Instead, we aim to provide you with many examples of techniques that we have used with our therapeutic groups in the hope that you will think about ways to create your own techniques suited to your particular population, your specific groups, and to you.

In designing your groups, you will certainly need to focus clearly on the basic goal you hope to attain. The time structure, the setting, the techniques you employ, the candidates you accept for the group, and your role as leader are all largely determined by the type of group you are designing. It is of central importance to consider the role techniques will play in the service of clients. In certain task groups, you may want to employ structured exercises and make use of a clear agenda that will guide your group sessions. If you are conducting a psychoeducational group for adolescents in a school, you may rule out certain techniques designed to bring about an exploration of intense emotions; these techniques are better suited to therapeutic groups. In creating and using techniques, therefore, you will always want to keep clearly in mind the primary purpose of your group. Techniques are tools to help you and your members accomplish that goal. Especially during the early stage of a group, certain techniques can help members clarify their goals.

In addition to a range of suggestions about recruiting, screening, informing, and preparing group members (see Chapter 3), we recommend a generic technique for virtually all groups. This consists of some form of invitation for members to declare their perception of the group, what they want from it, or something that will involve them in formulating the group's direction. Specific suggestions for these "check-ins" will be found throughout the book. We routinely ask group members at the outset of a workshop, a group course, or a session of an ongoing group to say something about what particular hopes, expectations, and fears they are bringing with them to the group.

In any given situation in a group, several different techniques can often be used, and each may be equally beneficial to a client. What basis does a leader have for choosing one technique rather than another? Leaders do well to consider factors such as their theoretical orientation, their level of training, the population that makes up the group, the personality of the individual member and the group leader, and the member's cultural context.

Theory as a basis. The theoretical persuasion of the group leader often dictates the selection of a technique. For example, free association by clients with minimal intrusion from the leader usually leads to regression and a re-experiencing of earlier memories. Asking clients to pay attention to what they are thinking and feeling as others are working tends to focus a person on the here-and-now. Techniques of reinforcement for behavior direct attention away from intrapersonal dynamics. Thus, the choice of techniques depends to some extent on the theoretical framework of the therapist.

In our group work, we tend to devise techniques that tap the thinking, feeling, and behaving dimensions of human experience. Each of the theoretical frameworks has a good deal to offer in providing strategies for creative work. At times, members can benefit from exploring their beliefs and assumptions, some of which may be self-limiting. At other times, they need to experience their feelings more deeply. Finally, members need to develop an action plan for translating their insights into new behaviors. The same person can profit from a different focus at various stages in his or her work.

In working with group members, we emphasize the *thinking* dimension. We typically assist members in thinking about the decisions they have made about themselves. We stress paying attention to "self-talk." How are members' problems actually caused by the assumptions they make about themselves, about others, and about life? How do members create their own problems by their thoughts and beliefs? In other words, many of our group techniques are designed to tap members' thinking processes, to help them think about events in their lives and how they have interpreted these events, and to work on a cognitive level to change certain belief systems.

We also value approaches that emphasize helping members identify and express their *feelings*. In the groups we lead, members often are stuck due to unexpressed and unresolved emotional concerns. If allowed to experience the range of their feelings and talk about how certain events have affected them, their healing process is facilitated. If members feel listened to and understood, they are more likely to express feelings they were unaware of or have kept to themselves.

As you will see in the many case examples presented in this book, group members can benefit from an emotional catharsis (the release of pent-up feelings), but some kind of cognitive work is also essential if the maximum benefit is to be gained. Both thinking and feeling need to be addressed.

A *behavioral dimension* is essential if the goal is behavior or personality change. Members can spend countless hours gaining insights and expressing pent-up feelings, but at some point they need to get involved in an action-oriented program of change. Bringing feelings and thoughts together by applying them to real-life situations focused on current behavior is emphasized by many of the cognitive behavioral approaches. If the focus of group work is on what people are doing, chances are greater that they will also be able to change their thinking and feeling.

Underlying our integrated focus on thinking, feeling, and behaving is our philosophical leaning toward the existential approach, which places primary emphasis on the role of choice and responsibility in the therapeutic process. In our groups we facilitate members' awareness of the choices they *do* have, however limited they may be, and encourage them to accept responsibility for choosing for themselves. Most of what we do in our groups is based on the assumption that people can exercise their freedom to change a situation or at least to change their response to it. Thus, we encourage members to focus on what they are thinking, feeling, and doing rather than attempting to change others. This integrative model of group work is described in detail in *Theory and Practice of Group Counseling* (Corey, 2004, chaps. 16 & 17).

Client population as a basis. Your sensitivity to the population with whom you are dealing is manifested in the techniques used. One cannot use the same techniques with a group of hospital patients that one would use with clients in a growth group. Similarly, techniques that tend to bring strong emotions to the surface need to be used cautiously with a group for people considered to be criminally insane. Techniques used for group therapy clients may be inappropriate for professionals such as nurses or teachers in a group for developing interpersonal skills. There is an almost limitless variety of groups, and a leader needs to ask: "What is the goal and purpose of the group? Is this technique suitable for this group of people? Is it the best available technique for this population in this situation?"

Client personality as a basis. A technique needs to be chosen with the personality of the individual group member in mind. If it does not fit, it most likely will not lead to productive work. Imagine asking a reserved elderly person to beat a pillow as an expression of her anger. Although the therapist may feel it valuable for her to express her anger, it is equally important to respect her ability and willingness to express anger in this fashion. There needs to be a congruence of the technique, the person introducing it, and the person for whom it is intended.

Adapting group techniques to the client's cultural context. In choosing techniques, it is essential to consider the ways in which the client's cultural background influences his or her personality and values. If a technique goes against the grain of a member's personality and culture, it will probably result in alienating the client from the group. The key is to present techniques in a way that respects the uniqueness of an individual's personal and cultural context.

If you expect to lead groups with culturally diverse populations, it will be essential that you discover ways to modify your strategies to meet their needs. Perhaps your genuine respect for the differences among members in your groups and your willingness to learn from them will be the most important foundation on which to build a bridge between yourself and them. It is particularly critical to monitor your own behavior so that you will avoid making stereotyped generalizations about individuals within a particular social or cultural group.

It is the responsibility of leaders to inform potential members of the values that will guide group interaction. For instance, these values may include staying in the here-and-now, expressing feelings, asking for what one wants, being direct and honest, sharing personal material with others, learning how to trust, improving interpersonal communication, learning to take the initiative, dealing with conflict, being willing to confront others, and deciding for oneself. Some of the values generally associated with group participation may not be congruent with the cultural norms of some clients. For example, some individuals might have difficulty being direct because their culture frowns on directness. Other clients may experience trouble putting themselves in the central place or taking up group time, largely because they have learned from their culture that to do so is rude and insensitive. Some members will not be comfortable making decisions for themselves without considering their extended family. Although some group techniques are designed to assist members in more freely expressing their feelings, certain members will find this offensive. Because of their cultural conditioning, certain individuals are averse to expressing emotions openly or to talking freely about problems within their family. They may have been taught that it is good to withhold their feelings and that it is improper to display emotional reactions publicly.

The ASGW (1998) guidelines specify that ethical practice requires that leaders be aware of the multicultural context in group work, as can be seen in this recommendation regarding group practice:

> Group Workers practice with broad sensitivity to client differences including, but not limited to ethnic, gender, religious, sexual, psychological maturity, economic class, family history, physical characteristics or limitations, and geographic location. Group Workers continuously seek information regarding the cultural issues of the diverse population with whom they are working both by interaction with participants and from using outside resources.*

Cultural diversity affects the issues that members bring to a group and the ways in which they might be either ready or reluctant to explore these issues. Group leaders need to sensitize themselves to the clues that members often give indicating that they would like to talk about some aspect of how their culture is affecting their participation in the group.

*Quotations in this book are from "Best Practice Guidelines," by the Association for Specialists in Group Work. Copyright 1998 by the ASGW. This and all other quotations from this source are reprinted by permission. Consult Appendix A for a copy of the current ASGW (1998) "Best Practice Guidelines."

It is possible to create techniques that give members an opportunity to talk about certain aspects of their culture. Several examples come to mind. One group member, Ramon, had a difficult time with a female co-leader who tended to be very direct and say exactly what was on her mind. His culture had conditioned him to use more indirect ways of communicating. Ramon had particular difficulty with a woman speaking her mind with such candor. In his culture women were supposed to be quiet and unassertive, and it was not appropriate for a woman to confront a man. Ramon also experienced problems with assertive women outside the group, and he let the leader know that he did want to talk about this situation. Another member, Rosalie, wanted an opportunity to let others in the group know that she had a hard time letting others take care of her. Her culture had reinforced her behavior of taking care of all her brothers and sisters, but it had not reinforced her for asking for others to nurture her. She had difficulty letting others in the group give to her, and she devoted much of her energy to taking care of members in the group who expressed pain. Both Ramon and Rosalie expressed a desire to question some of their cultural upbringing and felt that they were better understood after they had had a chance to let others know what their culture had taught them and how these lessons were affecting their behavior in the group. Once they felt that others understood their cultural frame of reference, it was possible to introduce techniques that would accentuate selected cultural themes and help these members decide whether they might want to modify some of their behavior.

We highlight cultural material as it emerges in a group session by providing individuals with an invitation to identify relevant dimensions of their culture. We might suggest any of the following:

- Tell us something about your culture and how you think it may influence your participation in this group.
- If you think some members of this group might have a certain cultural perspective different from your own, would you pick out some of these members and tell each of them about some of the things that you are likely to see differently?
- Could you pretend for a moment that you're home among members of your ethnic group? Try to explain to them what this group is all about. What would you say?

The point of techniques of this kind is to bring certain cultural material to the surface so that misunderstandings or potential conflicts can be dealt with openly. If these themes remain latent, unspoken thoughts and unexpressed reactions are likely to interfere with the development of cohesion. Although members do share some universal human concerns, the members are also different from one another. Likewise, members of the same culture can be different. A group is an ideal place for people to learn how to understand, appreciate, and respect their cultural differences at the same time as they discover ways in which they are bonded by common concerns.

Introducing Techniques

Learn to pay attention to how you introduce techniques. To what extent do you explain them? How do you ask members to participate in them? How do you work with members who are reluctant to follow your suggestions? Let's discuss each of these questions in some detail.

Explaining techniques. You cannot always explain a proposed technique, the rationale for its use, and the desired outcome in detail prior to its use. To do so may render the technique useless. For instance, a lengthy explanation may interrupt the flow of the material. Or an explanation that specifies an anticipated emotion—"You'll probably experience a lot of pain and cry if you do this"—may set the client up to artificially display that feeling or to talk about it. We do not usually try to explain the outcome to our groups. For example, a woman says she may be too critical. It may be effective to introduce an exercise that encourages her to be critical, based on our hunch that being critical is indeed a part of her. Then it is possible to leave it to the process to prove whether our hunch is correct. Part of the preparation of group members should include a general discussion about techniques and how they serve the purpose of a group.

Inviting members to participate. It is our practice to invite group members to go along with a technique and to proceed only when we sense that we have their permission. We tend to use such phrases as these: "Are you willing to take this further?" "Are you willing to try this?" "I have something in mind that might help you understand better what you are saying. Let me tell you what it is, and see whether you are willing to go along with it."

An invitational stance both offers respect and encourages group members to challenge their values and behaviors. If we are working with Brian, a client who is ethnically different from us, we make room for the fact that his differences might partially account for behavior in the group that could be perceived as "resistance." For example, he may be very quiet yet observant in the group, and he may seek advice from us about what would be the right course for him to take in coping with his problems. We do not quickly assume that he is resistant and dependent. Instead, we pursue with him the possible meanings of certain of his behaviors. In doing so, we may learn that he is silent because he has learned that this is a sign of respect. His culture may have taught him not to put the focus of attention on himself. Also, his conditioning may prime him to seek direction from people he considers authorities. By respectfully gathering data about Brian with his help, we are in a better position to teach him ways to get what he needs from the group without violating his cultural norms.

Working with clients' reluctance. If group members say that they are not willing to participate in an exercise, we might ask "Are you willing to talk about your hesitation?" If the answer is still negative, we usually let it go. If clients develop a style of declining invitations to work, we point it out to them and ask if they are interested in doing anything about this pattern. Clients should not be harassed or pushed into doing what they are unwilling to do, but members need to be challenged if a group is to get work done.

Note that we ask our clients to talk about why they do not want to go along with what we suggest. This is a genuine request, and we do not automatically label their behavior resistance. Their resistance may be because we have missed something important about them, as in Brian's case, which is a good illustration of how we can work with what appears to be a member's reluctance to participate in a respectful, yet challenging, manner.

Much "resistance" is justified caution on the part of the client. Most often members are willing to talk about their reluctance, and almost inevitably this discussion leads to important issues for the group, such as the trust or distrust felt toward certain members or perhaps toward the leader. If such issues arise, the sensitive leader abandons the technique, perhaps introducing a different technique appropriate for pursuing the theme of lack of trust. For example, the leader might now say something like this: "I would like to be able to work with you, but I'm having trouble knowing how to proceed. You've indicated that you don't feel safe in here yet, and that perhaps explains your reluctance to go along with some of the exercises. I hope that you're willing to talk about what it would take for you to feel more trusting in here. Would you be willing to say something to each person in this group, myself included, that makes it easy or difficult for you to feel trust?" This technique can lead to good outcomes for the group, increased cohesion, and willingness in the future to go along with suggested techniques.

In a Nutshell

In this section we highlight a series of points that clarify some of the underlying principles of why we lead the way we do. As group practitioners, we draw upon concepts and techniques from most of the contemporary therapeutic models and adapt them to our own unique personalities. As mentioned earlier, our conceptual framework takes into account the *thinking, feeling,* and *behaving* dimensions of human experience.

We want to emphasize that these are our views and that we are presenting them for you to consider and to adapt for yourself in a way that makes sense to you. These are not pronouncements about the best way to lead a group, but they are ideas that have worked well for us. As such, we recommend them for your consideration.

Recognize the primacy of the client. In this book we may seem more directive and structured in our leadership style than is really the case. Although we take an active role in leading, we are constantly responding to our clients and taking clues from them. We see therapy as a kind of dance: sometimes we lead and sometimes we follow, but in either case we try to be aware of how we can best move with our partners. Sensitivity to and respect for clients are fundamental to the therapeutic interaction. We seek to suit techniques to clients rather than molding them to our needs and our techniques.

Realize the importance of preparation. It is a good practice to prepare both yourself and the members for a group experience. Adequate preparation reduces the risks of group work and maximizes effectiveness. Preparation includes informing potential members about the nature of the group, teaching them about how they might get the most from a group experience, and encouraging them to focus on the specific issues and concerns they wish to explore. You can get yourself psychologically ready for a group by taking time to reflect on your own life and to think about your objectives for the group. Preparing with a co-leader whom you can learn from and who complements your own style can be ideal.

Emphasize confidentiality. Group participants are not going to reveal themselves in meaningful ways unless they feel quite sure that they can trust both you and the other members to respect what they share. One of your key responsibilities as a group leader is to protect members by defining clearly what confidentiality means and helping them understand the difficulties involved in maintaining it. Of course, the limitations of confidentiality need to be clarified at the outset, such as those situations in which you are legally obliged to divulge confidences. At appropriate times throughout a group, you might remind the members how crucial maintaining confidentiality is to their effective work.

Although members will inevitably want to talk about their group experiences with significant people in their life, it is wise to caution them about the subtle ways in which they might unintentionally violate others' confidences in this process. As a general rule, members do not violate confidentiality when they talk about *what* they learned about themselves in a group. They tend to get into trouble when they begin to talk about *how* others made changes by describing what others did or what techniques were used.

Use techniques as means, not ends. Techniques are no better than the person using them and are no good at all if they are not sensitively adapted to the particular client and context. The outcome of a technique is affected by the climate of the group and by the relationship between therapist and client. Techniques are a means to an end; they amplify material that is present and encourage exploration of where that material is leading. If you become more concerned with techniques than with what is best for the members, or if techniques become ends in themselves, positive group outcomes are jeopardized.

Cultivate the soil. Techniques should not be sprung on group members or be imposed without regard for the degree to which a relationship with the members has been cultivated. Particularly with techniques that evoke emotions, we think it is important to gauge the readiness of the client to work with us and with the exercise we are proposing. Instead of commanding, we invite clients to experiment with new behavior. It is our task to earn their trust by demonstrating our goodwill.

Use tentative language. We characteristically introduce a technique by saying "I wonder whether you would be willing to _______?" "How would it be if you _______?" or "Do you suppose you could _______?" When we offer an interpretation, we typically begin with phrases such as "I have a hunch that . . ." or "If I were you, I might feel that. . . ." We try in our choice of words not to give the impression that we know exactly what is going on. It is important, however, not to water our words down with meaningless qualifiers. We give our own confrontive feedback, for example, in a more direct and unqualified way. But in providing interpretations and in introducing techniques, we employ tentative language that gives the client room to gracefully decline.

Use simple language. Introduce techniques in a simple and clear manner. Groups inevitably develop their own special language and metaphors, but we tend to discourage using overworked popular expressions and psychobabble such as "getting in touch with your feelings." We strive to use language that is clear and descriptive.

Encourage verbalization. A great many of our techniques emphasize verbal behavior: role playing, sentence completions, and go-arounds. This emphasis fits with our theoretical commitment to thinking, feeling, and doing as a package, because what we say reveals how we think, feel, and act. Typically, when we ask group members to say something, we hope to promote their talking spontaneously, making their internal rehearsals known to others. Internal ruminations that are harshly judged by an individual are often met with acceptance and respect by others in the group.

Be aware of nonverbal communication. Be conscious of the nonverbal communications of group members and of how you nonverbally present yourself to the group. To establish a trusting relationship, we choose our words to communicate a basic respect for the people we work with. We recognize the importance of paying attention not only to the content of a member's speech but also to the manner in which the client presents messages. We look for patterns of nonverbal communications, yet we generally avoid quickly interpreting the meaning underlying these messages. Instead, we ask clients to become aware of their own body language and other nonverbal forms of communication and to attach their own meanings to patterns that emerge within the group. However, a caution is in order. It can become annoying to group members if leaders continually point out a person's particular body language or overly attribute meaning to nonverbal gestures.

Put aside prejudices and assumptions. If you want to be a therapeutic agent, we think it is essential that you put aside your preconceived notions about the people with whom you work. It is critical that you develop an awareness of the negative impact of stereotyping individuals because of their age, disability, ethnicity, gender, race, religion, or sexual orientation. Try to avoid making assumptions about clients. Be open to letting them tell you who they are and what is important to them. In this way you can avoid imposing your values and your vision of reality on clients who differ from you. Your techniques will certainly take into account factors such as the client's age and cultural background. For example, if you are working with adolescents and introduce a technique that assumes they feel rebellious, or if you are working with the elderly and introduce a technique that assumes they are no longer sexual, you are imposing your preconceived notions rather than allowing your clients to tell you who they are.

Adapt your techniques to the needs of culturally diverse clients. Culture does influence a client's behavior, whether or not the group counselor is aware of it, and responsible and effective practice entails an understanding of the range of cultural similarities and differences. It is useful to consider culture from a broad perspective that includes factors such as ethnicity, family traditions and beliefs, religion, race, socioeconomic status, and gender. Discover ways to modify your strategies to meet the unique needs of a group composed of culturally diverse members. Your genuine respect for the differences among members in your groups will be an important foundation on which to build a bridge between yourself and them. Effective multicultural practice calls for an open stance on your part and a flexibility in adapting your techniques to fit the needs and situations of the individuals within the group. No one "right" set of techniques can be utilized across the board, irrespective of a client's cultural background.

Be aware of values. Techniques are an extension of you as a person, but they must fit the context and the character of the client as well. It is not possible for your own values, which are a part of your character, to be excluded entirely from the material you pursue and the techniques you suggest. Strive to develop an awareness of how your values and needs are likely to influence the interventions you make. Although ethical practice dictates that you take care to avoid imposing your values on members, it may be appropriate that you express your beliefs and values in cases where concealing them is likely to create problems for those who participate in your groups.

Generally, we take our cues from what our clients indicate they want for themselves. When our own values come into play, we feel that at least we can be aware of them in ourselves. If a value of yours is that conflict should be avoided at all costs, you are likely to introduce techniques that bypass conflict. If a value of yours is that anger needs to be expressed, you are likely to develop techniques for dealing with the expression of anger. Minimally, you can be aware of your preferences and can make yourself and your values known to clients. In that way you are not as likely to use your preferences to manipulate others.

Present the problem to the group. Group leaders often wonder how to handle a situation and fail to utilize the most obvious resource: the wisdom of the group members. One of the simplest ways to get good help from the members is to ask for it; present the problem to them. For instance, if we are trying to think of a technique that might enhance a member's direction or are wondering how to modify a technique that is going nowhere, we may simply state the problem as we see it to the group and ask for suggestions. These interjections do double duty: they serve as interpretations or clarifications, and they constructively involve the group members in the process of seeking solutions.

Don't fight the river. We may sometimes introduce a technique thinking we know what is going to happen, but the material that emerges may lead in another direction. Or a client may misunderstand our directions and do something quite different from what we had in mind. We also find that a technique may work well once or many times, but we cannot always count on its working the same way twice. There are times when we have a sense of what we would like to introduce into a session, such as a focus on a particular theme or topic, yet the group may show little interest in pursuing our agenda. In all these instances, we prefer not to fight the river.

Be willing to experiment. In some ways the difference between an experienced leader and an inexperienced one lies in not being afraid to experiment and to forge ahead. We depend on our emotional and cognitive resources in creating techniques to fit a context. We teach beginning group leaders to be aware of certain pitfalls and to take necessary precautions, but we equally seek to encourage them to trust themselves. If you find yourself becoming stale or uncreative, you might consider getting more supervision, working more with different co-leaders, or attending different sorts of workshops as a participant.

Be willing to seek consultation. There will be times when you can profit from the input of colleagues or supervisors. Ethical practice involves the willingness to seek appropriate professional assistance when you become aware that your own personal problems or conflicts are likely to impair your professional judgment and your work with clients. Additionally, it is a mark of professionalism to seek out consultation or supervision regarding ethical concerns when you encounter difficulties that interfere with your effectiveness in carrying out leadership functions.

Realize that personal counseling may be called for. As a group counselor, you should recognize that exploring your own life is an ongoing process. You probably cannot, and, in any case should not, take your clients any further than you yourself are willing to go. Remain open to seeking personal counseling at times in your life when you are unable to work through a personal difficulty or crisis. Personal therapy is called for when your unresolved problems prevent you from being as effective as you might be.

Link the work of clients. For group techniques to be most effective, they generally ought to allow for several members to work at the same time. Some individual work in a group setting can be fine, but involving several clients better utilizes time and resources. In this area the leader orchestrates the group using creativity and intuition to identify common themes from the information clients have provided and to indicate how members can work together on these themes.

Use the client's metaphors. We try to follow the lead provided by our group members' material and we see techniques as a means of enhancing what is going on rather than trying to generate a direction according to our own agenda. A key aspect of this view is that we design techniques that utilize the phrasings and metaphors introduced by the group member. The member's language finds its way into our ideas for techniques, and it provides us with the occasion for creative work.

In supervising student group leaders, we find that, out of anxiety, they often focus on the client's literal message. They may not "hear" the member's metaphor, or if they do, they often miss the rich source of meaning contained in it. For example, when members say that they feel empty inside, it is therapeutically useful to look beyond the literal by encouraging them to explore what emptiness means to them. How do they describe emptiness? How do they experience emptiness? If they feel empty, what may they be missing? What are they inclined to do with this feeling?

Consider the richness of these metaphors: "I feel that I have a hole in my soul." "I am surrounded by walls." "I feel like the only fire hydrant on a street with five dogs." "I am a bottomless pit." "I feel like a doormat." Any of these symbols can speak volumes about the experience of a member. For instance, it is therapeutically useful to pursue the person's experience of being a "doormat." Members seldom realize the depth of their metaphors, and leaders need to tune into that.

Use humor. Humor can be used to deflect painful or uncomfortable situations in a group, but if used appropriately and timed well, it can be therapeutic. We are struck by how clients can laugh about topics they were crying over only a short time before. We don't hesitate to have fun and to make humor part of the techniques we introduce. For genuine and constructive humor to be used in a group there has to be a strong level of trust. Furthermore, humor should never be used to denigrate a member. In a climate of respect, the humor involves laughing *with* members, not at them. Again, let us stress that humor is not to be used to avoid serious work.

Go with the obvious. Although we may use interpretations as a way of thinking about our clients, we work with what is present and obvious. When a group seems flat, you might be tempted to assume responsibility by using techniques to "get the group going." Rather than trying to bring energy to the group, we suggest that you call attention to what is obvious to you and describe what you see to the members. Describing what you see without judgment or labeling is very respectful of what the members are experiencing and cannot express.

Think about theory. We emphasize the importance of continually rethinking our theoretical orientations. A theory is a cognitive map, but not a fixed map. Our theories about how to work are open to modifications based on experience. We try to be aware of how we are viewing human nature and how this view affects our style of therapy, what our rationale is for introducing the techniques we do, and what our vision is of what we have to offer clients. Some practitioners have a high regard for their intuitions and hunches but downplay the intellect and are unwilling to reflect on what they are doing. Leaders must be willing to review their theoretical assumptions if their techniques are to be meaningful.

Recognize the limits of responsibility. We see the therapeutic partnership as an opportunity to examine our lives, our feelings, and our possibilities for being different. Earlier, we used the metaphor of therapy as a dance, in which the therapist sometimes leads, sometimes follows, but always seeks to go with the shared movement. Responsibility for the success of the dance is not ours alone. We see our responsibilities primarily as preparing ourselves and our members for the group experience, providing a context in which meaningful work is possible, making ourselves available to hear and encounter our clients, providing skills and techniques that facilitate the explorations of the group, and seeking to maximize the opportunity to learn from the experience. If a group goes well, it is not all to our credit, and if a group is unproductive, it is not all our fault.

Don't attempt to change people directly. We assume that our clients may change under our influence, but we don't see these changes as something we do to them as if they, like the sculptor's clay, were the passive recipients of our technical manipulations. We do not think that people's lives simply and passively undergo transformation as a result of what we do. We seek to provide an optimal environment, or context, within which group participants can reexamine and rethink decisions they have made, express what they feel, try out new behavior, and, in short, consider how they could change. Although a technique we introduce can invite participants to change and encourage them to do so, we do not think it is the technique that brings the change about. The technique simply enhances the client's awareness of the possibility of being different. Once the client is aware of these options, the hardest work begins as the client attempts to carry what has been learned into daily life.

Attempt to integrate thinking, feeling, and doing. People cannot be segmented, because thinking, feeling, and acting are necessarily interdependent. One dimension of human functioning invariably affects other aspects of behavior. Thus, our techniques work better when we strive to utilize all modes of experience. If we sometimes ask clients to refrain from thinking about what they are saying, our goal is to have them eventually think clearly and be in a position to change. Some theories of therapy emphasize feeling as opposed to thinking; some stress thinking rather than feeling; some accentuate behavior independently of thinking or feeling. We emphasize the integration of these three dimensions. We seek through our use of techniques to give our clients an opportunity to experience and express their emotions. But we are also concerned to have them reflect on how their feelings connect with their belief systems, the assumptions they make, and the early decisions on which these assumptions may be based. We focus considerably on what they are currently doing, realizing that their actions are influenced by what they are thinking and feeling. Then we encourage them to try out different ways of behaving within the group and, lastly, to consider ways of carrying concrete behavioral changes into their lives outside the group.

Explore polarities. To achieve our goal of integrating thinking, feeling, and doing, we seek to acknowledge and work with polarities in our clients. All clients have opposite sides within them, even though they often do not want to acknowledge or own them: a thinking side versus a feeling side, being like one parent versus being like the other, being dependent versus being independent, being passive versus being active, being trusting versus being suspicious, and being open versus being closed. Many of our techniques ask group members to exaggerate one side of themselves to get more information about it and to decide whether it is a way they want to be. Our techniques do not aim at getting rid of one side. Rather, we find that having clients acknowledge various sides of themselves through techniques that emphasize polarities is a prelude to their accepting parts of themselves that they have needlessly rejected, rejecting parts they have needlessly accepted, and considering possibilities for integrated change.

Work with the past, present, and future. Some leaders think of their groups as having a present, or here-and-now, orientation. Others focus on the past based on the premise that the past influences present choices. Still others emphasize the direction we are moving toward, or a future orientation. The groundwork for change involves helping clients clearly understand who they are now based on their personal histories. Our techniques move back and forth among all three temporal frames of reference. Typically, we begin with current concerns introduced by group members and with dynamics we see in the group. We assume that present material is rooted in childhood lessons, but when we introduce techniques that focus on the past, we seek to use only material that can be made experientially present. We also operate on the assumption that if we focus on the client's present state, this person's unfinished business from the past will become evident.

There are themes in a person's life, and we are interested in seeing connections between one's past and one's current personality. To make the past more relevant and to explore it in a more lively way, we frequently ask clients to bring their past into the present by imagining and reliving significant scenarios. We may ask: "If you could be that hurt child you were then, what would you want us to know about you? What would you want from us?" or "What do you want to say to your father now that you didn't say then?" We avoid exploring past history in an abstract and detached way. We seek to examine the relevance of the past by reliving it and connecting it with current struggles. The point of such techniques is to put clients into a position to choose how they want to be now in light of their beginnings.

Provide opportunities to consolidate learning and to practice new behavior. The final stage of a group presents an ideal opportunity for using techniques that enable members to remember the specifics of their group experience, to seek a cognitive framework for lessons they want to take away, and to practice new behavior. Ideally, if the group is to be more than a passing experience, the group leader will promote consolidation, generalization, and transfer of learning.

Concluding Comments

The key point of this chapter is that techniques are valuable and important but must be used with caution. Because of the immediate progress that techniques seem to promote, the therapist may draw on them mechanically or may fail to explore material that they bring out. Techniques should be chosen in and for the situation; they are not to be memorized and then imposed on the group process. Our main concern in this book is not to equip you with an arsenal of group strategies but to encourage you to design techniques that are extensions of yourself, your own sensitivities, and the work of the member. We certainly are not urging you to memorize the techniques discussed here. Instead, we hope you use this book as a tool for improving your own ability to devise techniques and to think through the rationale for and the possible consequences of the techniques you invent.

Questions and Activities

At the end of each chapter we provide some questions and activities that we hope you will use to clarify your own positions and to integrate what you have read. We list far more questions and activities than we think any one person will be interested in pursuing in depth. We encourage you to read all the questions and then select the ones that have the most interest and value for you, modifying them to match your own interests, client population, and situation. If you are using this book as a classroom text, many of the questions and activities can be adapted for small group discussion, role playing, essay questions, and debates. The activities can be tried out in experiential groups.

Here are some questions and activities related to the discussion of topics in this chapter.

1. How would you define a technique? What is your view of the role that techniques should ideally play in the group process?
2. As a group leader, to what extent do you use techniques, and when do you think it is appropriate or inappropriate to do so? How does your use of techniques fit with your overall view of what a group is for?
3. We take the position that there are more important factors in group work than techniques. If you agree, what do you think these factors are? If you disagree, explain your position.
4. What do you think about approaching a group with a strict agenda rather than letting the group take its own course? Give an example of a population for which an agenda might be appropriate.
5. What are your ideas about using planned group exercises and techniques as a means of stimulating interaction in a group?
6. Give some examples of how and when techniques might interfere with the group process.
7. What are some ways in which you can adapt your techniques to fit the needs of the culturally diverse clients who are likely to be in your groups? How can you create techniques that will accommodate the differences among clients rather than forcing these clients to fit a predetermined technique? Think of some examples of how you might be inflexible in using techniques with culturally diverse populations.
8. As a group leader, to what degree do you see yourself as structuring and directing the groups you lead, and how would your employment of techniques reflect this structure?
9. We spoke of the importance of the relationship between leader and client. Can this relationship be obscured through the use of techniques?
10. What is your understanding of resistance? Do you see resistance simply as something to be gotten around? Why or why not? Do you see resistance as unwillingness to work? How would you work with resistance?
11. When and how could you explain to a client your rationale for suggesting a technique?
12. Have you participated in a group as a member? What did this experience teach you about yourself? about the group process? about leading groups? How might it help you or hinder you if you had no group experience?
13. What are some ways in which you can best learn which techniques are appropriate and which best fit your personality?
14. In this chapter (see "In a Nutshell") we have described key aspects of our philosophy of the place of techniques in group counseling. What three key points most interested you?

15. ***Challenges Facing Group Leaders* (DVD and Workbook).** Here are some suggestions for making effective use of this first chapter along with the first segment of *Challenges Facing Group Leaders,* the second program in *Groups in Action.*
    (a) As you view this second program, what characteristics do you observe in this group that illustrate difficult turning points in a group? In general, how would you describe the techniques used by the Coreys?
    (b) The Coreys view their task as intervening in a way that makes the room safe and provides a climate whereby members can talk about their hesitations and any resistance they may be experiencing. What is the importance of carefully working with whatever members bring to a group regarding their fears, concerns, or reservations? How is this kind of exploratory work essential if you hope to help a group move to a deeper level of interpersonal interaction? From reading this chapter and viewing the first segment of *Challenges Facing Group Leaders,* what are you learning about techniques to effectively work with members?
    (c) As you watch and study segment one (*Challenges of Dealing with Difficult Behaviors in Group*), notice signs of problematic behaviors on the part of members. Also notice signs of defensiveness and reluctance and how members express and work with their resistance. The themes that are enacted in segment one of this video program are illustrative of challenges that group leaders typically encounter in many different groups. These themes include the following:
        - Checking in: What was it like to return to group?
        - The leaders let me down.
        - I'm not feeling safe in here.
        - I didn't want to come back to group.
        - I'm in this group against my will.
        - Emotions make me uncomfortable.
        - I'm self-conscious about my accent.
        - I want the leaders to disclose more.
        - I learn a lot by being quiet.
        - Silence serves a function.
        - I feel pressured to disclose.
        - What's wrong with helping others?
        - Can't we stop all this conflict?
        - I feel weak when I show feelings.
        - Checking out: What are each of you taking from this session?
    (d) In small groups, explore these questions: What kind of difficult group member would present the greatest challenge to you? Do you have any ideas about why a certain problematic member might "trigger" you more than others? What do you see the co-leaders doing when members display behaviors that could be seen as problematic? What lessons are you learning about how to work therapeutically with challenging behaviors of members? How would you describe the manner in which the Coreys use techniques?

CHAPTER TWO

Ethical Issues in Using Group Techniques

Introduction

Before turning to specific techniques, we would like in this chapter to discuss some ethical concerns about using techniques in group work, with a focus on their responsible use. The abuse of techniques does not always stem from a lack of concern for members; it can also arise from a lack of awareness of the potential effects of procedures. We do not attempt to address the broad ethical problems of group work in this chapter. Instead, we are concerned here mainly with specific ethical issues posed by the use of techniques:

- The group leader as a person, and how the personal and professional aspects of group leadership are related to ethical and competent group practice
- The leader's motivations and therapeutic stance (the possible misuse of techniques for personal reasons and the leader's rationale for the techniques employed)
- Group preparation and norms (providing members with information about the leader, the group's structure and function, and basic policies)
- Using techniques as avoidance devices (such as not dealing with members directly or omitting material with which the leader feels uncomfortable)
- Avoiding undue pressure (pressure from peers and leaders to participate, misuse of aggressive and confrontational techniques, forced touching, and inappropriate catharsis)
- Protecting members when physical techniques are used
- Competence in using techniques

We hope you will develop a level of competence and will trust yourself to devise techniques creatively. However, you need to strike a balance between this creativity and a healthy caution in using techniques. If you have a sound academic background, have had extensive supervised group experience, have acquired some skills in group work, have had your own therapy, and have a fundamental respect for your clients, you are not likely to abuse techniques. Specific knowledge about the group process and specific skills in facilitating groups are essential for effective and ethical practice of group work.

The Leader as a Person

We emphasize the leader's involvement in moving the group forward. In this regard, the leader's character, personal qualities, and philosophy of life are more important than any technique for facilitating the group process. As a group leader, you are more than the sum total of your skills. From this viewpoint, when you take from another source a technique that is not a reflection of your own character and style, you are introducing something that is alien to you. If you are a low-key person and you introduce a highly dramatic technique, chances are that the discrepancy will inhibit the group. You can, instead, use your unique personal qualities as a part of your therapeutic style. You may have a wit that can be used appropriately. Your playfulness and supportiveness can become an integral part of how you facilitate a group. Whatever personal dimension you draw from, it is critical to remember that in many ways the person you are is your best therapeutic instrument. Ethical behavior cannot be separated from the person that you are.

Some group leaders depend on techniques far too much to get out of difficult situations, to get groups moving, or to keep them moving, and in doing so they become mechanical facilitators. This practice ignores the most powerful resource for reaching group members: the leader's personal reactions to the members and to what is going on between group members.

Both the existential approach to groups and the person-centered approach to groups (see Corey, 2004, chaps. 9 & 10) place primary emphasis on the personal qualities of the group facilitator rather than on techniques of leading, because the main role of the facilitator is to create a healing climate in the group. Both of these approaches to groups put more emphasis on experiencing the group member in the present moment than on using a particular set of interventions. Technique follows understanding, which means that the primary concern of the group counselor is to be *with* the group member and to understand his or her subjective world. These theoretical orientations are based on the assumption that there are no "right" techniques, because the task is accomplished through the therapeutic encounter between members and the group facilitator.

It is important to acquire knowledge of how groups function, to learn the necessary skills and techniques to implement your knowledge in actual group work, and to do so in such a way that your techniques become an expression of your personal style and an extension of the unique person you are. We hope that you will take what we have to offer in these chapters to create your own variations—that you will develop a recipe that suits your taste. We are proposing an experimental attitude, and we encourage you to try out techniques and different ways of working in a group to gradually learn what works for you, as well as what does not.

How can you use techniques that are an extension of yourself as a person? We'd like to make some suggestions.

Pay attention to yourself. A good place to begin is by monitoring your own experience in the group, including looking at the impact you have on the members. This process involves assessing your level of investment, your directness, your willingness to model what you expect of your members, and your willingness to be psychologically present for them. How high is your own energy level and your own readiness to be responsive to the group? You will tune in to the group more sensitively if you are in the habit of tuning in to yourself.

Learn to trust yourself. Learning to trust yourself is another essential part of the task of finding a style that suits your personality. If you do not trust your hunches, you may hold yourself back from even trying certain techniques. One way to develop this kind of trust is by being willing to follow your hunches and by trying variations of the techniques we describe. If a technique does not work, the consequences do not have to be horrible. Simply acknowledging that an exercise or a technique is not working is often the best way of pulling yourself out of a situation that could otherwise become worse. It is not helpful to worry so much about making mistakes that you block yourself from making many interventions. If you believe you must be absolutely sure before you act, you will miss many opportunities for action, and your clients will be deprived of opportunities as well. It takes courage to admit that a particular intervention did not work. What is crucial to us is how we recover from mistakes.

Model. Another way to be sure that your use of techniques reflects your personality is through modeling. Modeling is not a technique to stir up feelings, but it can be a catalyst for members to get in contact with their experience largely through your example. You can invite members to broaden their range of group behavior by demonstrating certain behaviors yourself. You can teach directness through your own directness. You can encourage members to give sensitive and honest feedback to others by doing so yourself. If you model nonjudgmental confrontation in a way that shows your concern for the person being challenged, your group members will learn how to confront one another in the same fashion. And through your openness, you invite members to share what they are experiencing.

Disclosing to group members what you are experiencing in the group is generally appropriate. However, when it comes to disclosing your problems from outside of the group, it is essential that you have guidelines for when and how you engage in self-disclosure. You need to be clear about your motivations for revealing your own personal issues and you need to monitor the impact of this on the group. A potential danger is that you may end up expressing your personal concerns more often than any member of the group. Your self-disclosures should be relevant to what is going on in the group, and the time you take should not be at the members' expense. Your disclosures should facilitate self-exploration and interaction within the group rather than burdening the members with your personal problems.

Approaching group sessions with a sense of enthusiasm generates enthusiasm within the group. Your vitality and your being psychologically present for members are in themselves powerful modeling agents in getting groups to move. Your degree of aliveness and enthusiasm may be an index of the degree to which your groups are able to function in a vital way.

In summary, techniques have more impact if you are able to maintain a relationship based on trust with group members. Such trust is best created through the personal qualities that you project. In other words, techniques do not work in isolation from your personality and your relationship with members. You make a difference.

Know your values. A group leader's values are a basic part of who the leader is as a person. A central ethical issue in the practice of group counseling involves group leaders' awareness of their values and the potential impact these values have on the interventions they make in their group. Group counselors must consider when it might be appropriate to expose their beliefs, decisions, life experiences, and values. The key is that leaders exercise care to avoid short-circuiting the members' exploration. The leader's central function is to help members find answers that are congruent with their own values.

From our perspective, the leader's function is to challenge members to evaluate their behavior to determine how it is working for them, not to advise members on the proper course to adopt. If members come to the realization that what they are doing is not serving them well, they are more open to being challenged by the leader to develop alternative ways of behaving that will enable them to reach their goals. Group leader behaviors that are hallmarks of ethical, professional, and effective practice include (a) demonstrating acceptance of the person of the client; (b) avoiding responding to sarcastic remarks with sarcasm; (c) educating the members about group process; (d) being honest with members rather than harboring hidden agendas; (e) avoiding judgments and labeling of members, and instead describing the behavior of members; (f) stating observations and hunches in a tentative way rather than dogmatically; (g) letting members who display difficult behavior know how they are affecting others in a nonblaming way; (h) detecting their own countertransference reactions; (i) avoiding misusing their power; (j) providing both support and caring confrontations; and (k) avoiding meeting their own needs at the expense of the members.

The Leader's Motivations and Theoretical Stance

Becoming aware of motivations. We are concerned about leaders who might be tempted to use techniques to protect themselves, to meet their own needs for power or prestige, or to control the members of their groups. Group leaders who are unaware of their motivations may misuse techniques in various ways: They may apply pressure on certain clients to get them to perform in desired ways. They may use techniques to impress participants. They may steer a member away from exploring feelings and issues they personally find threatening. They may use highly confrontive techniques and exercises to stir up their members. In all such cases, the leader's needs become primary, while those of the members assume relative unimportance.

Even experienced leaders are sometimes slow to recognize their motivations in their use of various techniques. If these abuses become patterns, one can hope that they will show up in the leaders' own therapy or supervised sessions. Co-leaders can also point out these patterns. Members most likely will also notice this. If leaders do not have supervisors or co-leaders, it is advisable to make it a habit to review group sessions and stay alert to ways in which their own needs and motives may be getting in the way. Group leaders do have needs, and some of these needs are met through their work in facilitating a group. However, it is not acceptable for leaders to exploit members to meet these needs.

Dealing with the superhuman image. Group members often attribute exaggerated power and wisdom to leaders, and there is a temptation for leaders to be seduced by this. One way to avoid this is to be willing to explain the purpose of a suggested technique. Although it is distracting to explain regularly the point of a technique in advance, at times it might be appropriate for a member to ask about the general purpose of a technique. For instance, Ferdinand said he felt cut off and lonely in the group. When the leader requested that he go into the next room, Ferdinand asked for a reason. Instead of insisting that he "just do it," the leader supplied a brief explanation: "I'd like you to have some sense of what it would be like to accentuate your feeling of being cut off so that we can explore that." At this point the leader might not want to explain certain other reasons for using the technique. For instance, she might have a hunch that Ferdinand was typically sent out of the room as a child and that this exercise would bring back those feelings and allow connections between them and his current loneliness to emerge. This hunch would be sabotaged if explained at the beginning, but it might be explained afterward. Explaining techniques in this way tends to discredit the impression that leaders possess superhuman qualities. In general, as the trust among members increases, techniques can be used that are increasingly challenging.

Having a therapeutic rationale. Although leaders cannot always predict the exact outcomes of techniques, they can have some idea of how a technique is connected with the material of the moment and where it is supposed to take the member. A supervisor, colleague, or a group member might ask you questions such as these: "Why did you use that technique?" "What did you hope to gain from it?" It is a good practice for you to pose these questions to yourself prior to leading a group. We are not encouraging you to be so preoccupied with thinking about the rationale for a technique that you become timid, but being aware of the purpose of a technique can become second nature and does not have to be incompatible with the ability to follow a hunch spontaneously.

The rationale for using a technique needs to be rooted in the whole picture of what the client has revealed. Every effort should be made to remember key themes from different episodes in the client's work. For example, one week Bill talked about his fear of becoming involved in an intimate relationship. In another session he was uninvolved in the group; he sprawled in his chair and seemed about to fall asleep. During another meeting, he said that he felt he was being treated coldly by others in the group. Remembering these episodes, the group leader attempted to bring them together by inviting Bill to sprawl out and look sleepily around the room, saying to each member a whole sentence that started with "A way I keep myself removed from you is _______." In this example the leader had a rationale: he sought to connect already existing material with the direction the technique was likely to take.

Group Preparation and Norms

The ASGW's (1998) "Best Practice Guidelines" are a set of professional and ethical guidelines for group practitioners (see Appendix A for this document). Let's examine some of the issues raised in these guidelines as they relate to group preparation and group norms.

Providing information about the group. The ASGW's (1998) "Best Practice Guidelines" specify that group workers have the responsibility to provide a professional disclosure statement and to prepare members for a group. Examples of some of the information potential members have a right to expect as a basis for making an informed decision about whether to become a participant can be found in sections A6 and A7 of the guidelines.

The techniques appropriate for a group depend on its goals and on the qualifications of the leader. Prospective members and referring agencies need to be fully informed about these goals and qualifications. Group leaders should have had academic training in a discipline related to human behavior, in-depth personal therapy or a self-exploration experience, and extensive supervised group work. In addition, it is important that you have a realistic perspective on the limitations of your own training gained from evaluations of your abilities by supervisors and professionals.

In setting group goals and identifying proposed techniques, it is imperative that you be clear about the main purpose of the groups you are designing and facilitating. Your experiences as a member of a group can be most valuable in giving you a personal understanding of techniques you may want to introduce in the groups you lead. Although you may not have experienced every specific technique you intend to use, it does help that you have personally experienced the general procedures you want to employ.

Informed consent is essential to ethical practice. A primary ethical issue involves explaining to prospective members of your groups the kinds of techniques that you are likely to utilize. It would be unrealistic to try to explain every technique in advance, but you can inform group members about your style and orientation of leadership. Your techniques should match your level of training and experience in group work. It is a mistake to suppose that the mere possession of a relevant academic degree and a license guarantees that you are qualified for using any and all techniques. It is important for you to fully inform prospective group members about your qualifications to lead a particular group.

Some of these issues can be addressed in literature or advertising about the group. One of the best times to inform prospective members about the goals of the group and the training of the leader is during screening and interviewing, which we discuss in Chapter 3.

Using tape recordings and videotapes. Recording devices are commonly used as techniques for training purposes and for giving feedback to members. Professors who teach group courses need to exercise adequate caution in using these training techniques, such as emphasizing confidentiality and informing students as to who might have access to these recordings. For the sake of the protection of members' confidentiality, it is essential that both professors and group trainees exercise the greatest care in viewing and critiquing tapes. If trainees are permitted to take tapes home for individual viewing, confidentiality can easily be compromised. It is essential that no recordings be made without the knowledge and express consent of the members of the group. Members have a right to know why the session is being recorded or videotaped, what will become of the material, and how it will be used. If the tapes will be used for research or will be listened to or seen and critiqued by a supervisor and students in a practicum, the members have a right to be informed of this use and to decline participation in the taping, if they so wish.

Leaders often find it useful to videotape a group session and allow members to view the tape before the next session. It can be agreed that the tape will be used only by the group members and the leaders. Such a tape should be erased when it is no longer needed for teaching purposes. If recording devices are used in this way, it is a good policy to inform members that they can stop the machine whenever they feel it is inhibiting their participation.

Using Techniques as Avoidance Devices

Avoiding a member's confrontation. A client attempting to express a legitimate reaction to the therapist was asked by the therapist to talk to an empty chair and to direct his concerns to the chair rather than to the therapist directly. Such avoidance of dealing directly with a client raises an ethical issue about the therapist's willingness to have honest interaction with clients. It implies that clients have no legitimate issues with the group leader, that what they have to say is only neurotic transference.

In another interchange a client expressed anger toward the leader, and the leader responded, "I'm glad you can get your feelings out." Such a response is condescending and suggests that the leader is preserving self-esteem at the expense of encountering clients. Group leaders sometimes find that they are intimidated by members' anger, especially when it is directed toward them. They need to acknowledge this and not deny it. At times their interventions are geared to patching up conflict quickly or avoiding it altogether. For instance, after one angry exchange between two members, one student leader, Herbert, suggested that the two embrace and exchange "positive feelings" instead of putting each other down. In essence, he asked them to pretend that the conflict did not exist rather than to explore what it was about. As a result of Herbert's discomfort, they did not get to the real issues between them. During the processing time, we focused on Herbert's discomfort over any display of anger or conflict. He readily admitted that in his family he had never been allowed to even feel anger, let alone express it openly. He was not clearly aware that the strategies he had introduced during the session were aimed at detouring the members' attempt to work through their conflict. As he talked about what he was feeling and thinking when he was leading, he was able to recognize how his personal limitations were influencing his ability to assist members in dealing with one another honestly.

As these examples show, when conflict exists within a group, it is essential that it be acknowledged directly and dealt with openly. The leader's techniques should not steer members away from what they are experiencing; rather, the techniques suggested are meant to facilitate direct interaction. If conflict is not brought into the open, it lies dormant and eventually inhibits productive work. Unrecognized conflict becomes a hidden agenda, which will certainly interfere with effective group interaction.

All too often in everyday life, people are conditioned to skirt the issue of facing and working through conflict. When conflict begins to brew in a group, the natural tendency is to quickly move it aside or to flee from it, but participants need to learn how to successfully work through their differences. Members can be challenged to try different behavior in a group setting by making a commitment to continue talking about their reactions to a conflict instead of avoiding the situation.

Avoiding the leader's fears. Group leaders need to guard against introducing techniques to cover up their own fear of exploring themes that are present in the group. Such diversion frequently occurs when there is distance or hostility in the group.

A student trainee, Pauline, was apparently upset over some unresolved conflict within the group. All of a sudden, she introduced a guided fantasy. Pauline asked members to close their eyes and take a few deep breaths and "just relax." She then guided them to recall a pleasant experience and to see themselves in a place where they very much liked to be. After about 10 minutes, one of the members, Sarah, finally exclaimed that she had to talk because she felt as if "I'm going out of my skin." As it turned out, Sarah was angry at Pauline, but she didn't feel that Pauline would allow her to deal with the source of her anger. Soon afterward, almost all of the members began talking about the hostility they had been feeling before Pauline's introduction of the guided fantasy that was aimed at relaxing them. As a result of processing what occurred during this session, the members finally began to open up and express reactions that they had been keeping hidden. This was a case where the wisdom of the group overrode the fear of the leader.

Genuine closeness in a group takes time to develop. During some periods in a group's history, closeness may be conspicuously absent. If leaders feel afraid, they may try to force a false sense of closeness through the use of various techniques. Suggesting that the members huddle together when they have expressed distance is not therapeutically sound. In this situation, it might be better to suggest that group members spread apart, to far corners of the room, and then talk about how they feel. In other words, leaders do well to strive to make explicit and even exaggerate what is already going on rather than trying to overcome their own fears by imposing an artificial solution.

A related abuse of techniques to avoid the leader's fear often occurs during awkward moments in groups. For example, the group may be lethargic, silences may be long, members may initiate little, and resistance may be manifested in several forms. At times like these we urge leaders to deal directly with this phenomenon. In an attempt to get things moving, some leaders may suggest an interaction technique or call on members directly and ask them questions. Resorting to such techniques in this situation is typically a manifestation of leader anxiety, and doing so often covers up potentially rich material.

A broad way of stating the ethical concern here is this: One of the most important things a group teaches is that we can learn to face and express what we think and feel. If we introduce techniques that detract from or cover up the dynamics of the group, we are modeling the idea that our feelings are something to be avoided.

In summary, one needs to be cautious about using techniques at all if they become substitutes for genuine exploration. In addition, when a technique is introduced, it is intended to highlight the cognitive, emotional, and behavioral material present in the group and not to detract from it because of the leader's unease.

Avoiding Undue Pressure

Freedom not to participate. Sometimes group leaders make use of interaction, communication, or nonverbal exercises to promote group interaction. For example, a leader may ask members to pair up and engage in a touching exercise or to otherwise express what they are feeling to their partners in a nonverbal way. If leaders are not careful, they can give the impression that all members are expected to participate in all these exercises. Members may feel pressured to do what everyone else is doing, but leaders must make it genuinely acceptable for them to pass by mentioning this option periodically whenever it is appropriate.

To avoid this problem, we usually invite members to work on personally meaningful material. If clients bring up issues they want to explore, the chances are increased that they can handle whatever might surface. Further, we typically impress on members that they can decide at what point they wish to stop. Clients sometimes open up a painful or threatening area and then say that they do not want to go ahead. Generally, we explore their desire for stopping, and in this way we can focus on the factors they find threatening. They may not trust the leader to deal with what they are facing. They may not trust the group enough to pursue an issue. They may be worried about looking foolish. Or they may fear losing control and not being able to regain composure. If members do decide to stop, we suggest that they tell us if they want to return to the issue later on. The responsibility is then clearly on the members to decide what they will bring out in the group and the depth to which they will explore the issues they do bring out. Placing responsibility on the members is a built-in safety factor, and it is a sign of our respect for them.

There is another side to this issue. We assume that people who come to a group require some challenge to work effectively. So the task is to achieve a balance between appropriate challenge and undue pressure (or unethical coercion). Leaders need to be alert to whether a client is leaving an opening for pursuing the technique, but they also have an ethical obligation to respect the client's refusal. We try to respect this refusal and yet explore the client's reasons for declining.

In these cases, much depends on the makeup and purpose of a given group, and even more depends on the relationship you have with a particular client. The more trust you have established with group members, and the more cohesive the group, the more you can challenge these members. The ethical issue centers on having a basic respect for working with material that is already present and, even more important, a basic respect for the client's decisions about what to explore and how far to go with it.

Pressure from other members. Group leaders have an ethical obligation to respond to undue peer pressure on a group member, especially when they have assured the group that no one will be coerced into making disclosures or participating in activities. The leader can comment on the peer pressure or can offer an interpretation of the seeming need to coerce and thus can turn the spotlight on the people exerting the pressure. The leader can ask them to talk about why they need to pressure someone else: "You seem intent on getting Jane to talk more. Would you tell her what makes this so important to you?" "Would you tell the group how you are going to feel if you fail to get Jane to do as you wish?" "Would it be relevant for you to talk about relationships you have had outside this group in which you wish someone would do what you are trying to get Jane to do?" The point of such interventions is to acknowledge the feelings of those who are exerting the pressure, and to see what productive work might be done with those feelings, while reminding the group of the need to respect the wishes of a reluctant member.

Misuse of confrontational techniques. At times group leaders can abuse their power by directing techniques toward a particular member. A group counselor opened a session by calling on a particular member, and he stayed with this person for the entire session. He believed this was an effective technique to use with resistant clients; he assumed that such pressure would break down their defenses. Although we think confrontational techniques can be used to work through members' resistances or defenses, we do have a problem with endless interrogation. When leaders resort to a barrage of questions, the members are likely to close themselves off. Other members tend to pick up the questioning behavior, the atmosphere of trust is lost, and clients are deprived of the opportunity to explore issues in depth. Instead, they think only about how to give appropriate answers to the questions thrown at them. Confrontation needs to be handled with care and concern for the member being confronted.

Forced touching. We do not discourage spontaneous touching in our groups, but we do not introduce a technique that explicitly directs clients into a physical intimacy that they do not want. As a group develops intimacy and takes risks, touching tends to increase, but then the touching has been earned rather than imposed. If two members are struggling to get to know each other and to break through their usual boundaries, a touching technique is only likely to bypass the hard work that meaningful intimacy requires.

Group counselors need to be cognizant that touching carries very different meanings for some group members. Depending on one's life experiences and one's cultural background, touching can have a variety of connotations. In some cultures, touching is avoided except with family members. For women and men who have been either physically or sexually abused, touching can recall negative feelings, even if it is done as an expression of concern. This is a topic that a group leader might want to introduce for discussion within the group so that no member's personal privacy is invaded.

An ethical issue of touching arises when a leader is asked to touch someone from whom he or she feels distant. Such a request may arise, for example, when the leader is role-playing a mother or father. Group leaders have an obligation to be genuine in such cases, partly because of the harm that dishonesty has already done to many of their clients. Here the ethical issue is that of being honest with clients and of modeling honesty and sensitivity. Clients are likely to sense when leaders are ignoring their own reservations. If leaders do not provide straight feedback, clients are deprived of an explanation for the lack of closeness in their lives.

Inappropriate catharsis. The success of a group is not measured by the degree of emotional intensity and cathartic experiences. Although the expression of emotion is an important component of the group process, the concern is in losing sight of what one hopes will emerge from catharsis. Moreover, group leaders and members can acquire the expectation that all members will display intense emotion and are somehow failures if they do not do so. We recall a group member who approached a leader during a break and said tearfully that she must not be getting anything from the group because she hadn't yet had a catharsis.

Among the ethical issues that catharsis involves are questions such as these: Whose needs are being met with the catharsis—those of the leader, the group, or the individual member? Is the leader clear about what the catharsis is supposed to mean or lead to? Is the leader capable of handling the intensity of the catharsis or what it might result in? Is there enough time in the group session to work with the emotions that arise and to arrive at a resolution? Will the group leader have subsequent sessions with the client to deal with potential repercussions of the catharsis? Is the leader sensitive to the subtle line between invoking catharsis for its therapeutic potential and invoking it for the sake of drama?

Leaders need to be especially aware of times when they use catharsis to fulfill their own needs and not those of their clients. A leader may want to see people express anger because she would like to be able to do so herself, and so she unethically pushes members to get into contact with angry feelings by developing techniques to bring out such feelings and to focus the group on anger. Techniques can also be developed that push members to express only positive and warm feelings toward one another. These are not illegitimate feelings, for surely most members are at times angry or feel close, but using techniques to exaggerate these feelings to satisfy the leader's needs is unethical. Group leaders need to ask this question frequently: "Whose needs are primary, and whose needs are being met—the members' or the leader's?"

Granting the freedom to leave. Some leaders contend that members always have the right to leave a group; others feel strongly that once members have committed themselves to a group they have an obligation to stay with it. The leader's attitudes and policies about this topic must be spelled out at a preliminary session.

Our position is that clients have a responsibility to the leaders and the other members of the group to explain why they want to leave. We have several reasons for this policy. It can be deleterious to members to leave without being able to discuss what they considered threatening or negative in the experience. In addition, it is unfortunate for members to leave a group because of a misunderstanding about some feedback they have received. On the other side, it can be damaging to other members if they suppose that someone left the group because of something they said or did. By having the person who is leaving present reasons to the group as a whole, other members have an opportunity to verify any concerns they may have about their responsibility for that person's decision.

We tell our members that they have an obligation to attend all sessions and to inform us, and the group, if they intend to miss a session or if they decide to withdraw. If members even consider withdrawing, we encourage them to say so, because such an acknowledgment inevitably provides extremely important material to explore in a session. Although we do not seek to subject members to a debate or to undue pressure to stay, we do stress the serious impact that their leaving will have on the whole group, especially if they do so without explanation. There may be times when a member wants to leave a group, even though the leader is convinced that doing so would not be beneficial for the client. In cases such as this, it is a good practice to offer the person a referral to another source of help.

Using Physical Techniques

Physical techniques, such as hitting pillows or arm wrestling, often have unpredictable outcomes. The symbolic release of aggression can be valuable, but certain precautions should be taken. Leaders who introduce such techniques must protect the client and the other members from harm, and they need to be prepared to deal with unforeseen directions that the exercise may take. The concern here is not simply for the physical safety of the clients. If a client has restrained emotion for a long time out of fear of the consequences of expressing it, that fear receives tragic reinforcement if the emotion does indeed get out of control when it is expressed and proves damaging to others. In general, we avoid physical techniques involving the whole group for reasons of safety.

Group counselors who introduce physical techniques should have enough experience and training to understand the process and possible consequences of such work. We encourage leaders to try techniques, but we also see a danger in their foolishly or unthinkingly using techniques that they have not experienced themselves or that easily generate material they have no idea how to handle. Merely reading about techniques and then trying them out is not sufficient. Beginning leaders should use them only when direct supervision is available or when they are co-leading with an experienced counselor.

In addition, as we stressed in the previous section, leaders must never goad or push members into physical techniques. Here, inviting members to participate in an exercise and giving them the clear option of refraining are essential. If leaders explain to members the exercise they have in mind, ask them whether they want to try it, and take safety precautions, the chances for negative outcomes are minimized. If physical techniques are occasionally used, it is essential to weigh the potential value of a technique against the potential risk. Besides the fact that group members can inadvertently be hurt, group practitioners may open themselves up to a malpractice suit through the use of physical techniques. In today's litigious society, leaders can make themselves legally and ethically vulnerable if they use certain physical exercises that could be misconstrued as harassment, sexual misconduct, or some other type of physical inappropriateness.

In using techniques, the central ethical issue is the competence of the leader, an issue we will address further in the next section. The leader who is not ready to deal with strong expressions of emotion ought not to be employing techniques likely to elicit them. A further concern is that the leader be sufficiently familiar with the client to have some basis for judging whether a technique that induces such catharsis is appropriate. These techniques should also be introduced when there is ample time, including follow-up time, for working through the material elicited. We prefer not to employ these techniques to introduce nonexistent feelings but only to work further with feelings that an individual client is already displaying and ready to intensify. Finally, we try to remember that growth can take place in thoughtful and reflective moments as well as in more overtly emotional situations, so we guard against using physical techniques out of a misplaced need for drama.

Competence in Using Group Techniques

Perhaps the most basic ethical issue pertaining to the use of group techniques is the level of competence achieved by the group leader. Group leaders should not use techniques for which they have not been trained or for which they are not under supervision by a counselor familiar with the intervention. A specific ASGW (1998) guideline (B.2) addresses the issue of possessing group competencies:

> Group workers have a basic knowledge of groups and the principles of group dynamics, and are able to perform the core group competencies, as described in the ASGW Professional Standards for the Training of Group Workers. Additionally, Group Workers have adequate understanding and skill in any group specialty area chosen for practice (psychotherapy, counseling, task, psychoeducation, as described in the ASGW Training Standards).

This issue is not as simple as determining whether someone is a competent group leader or an incompetent one. One needs to consider what competencies are required with what population and with what specific type of group. One way for you to keep up to date with your knowledge of techniques is to read the professional journals and selected books in group counseling. It is also crucial to do specialized reading about the various populations with which you are working. Simply completing a single course in group counseling as a part of a degree program will not ensure your competence in working with certain challenging populations. Training workshops can upgrade your group leadership skills.

Students who are in training with us frequently worry whether they know enough to effectively utilize a wide variety of techniques. Although we do not recommend the thoughtless use of techniques that could open up intensive work for members, we do encourage these trainees to experiment in a safe setting with techniques that are unlikely to lead to work too intense for them to handle. The first principle that we try to get across is the necessity for trainees to experience a wide range of techniques as a member of a group. Merely reading about a technique in a book, observing techniques being used by professionals, or simply discussing techniques does not equip trainees with the skills or the confidence to appropriately and effectively employ techniques. Because we are convinced of the value of certain kinds of experiential group work, we encourage our students to seek out groups in which they can participate fully as a member. This experience has proven invaluable, along with taking courses and getting supervision in training workshops.

Concluding Comments

The most important ethical point we have made in this chapter is that techniques can be harmful if used inappropriately or insensitively. They can injure group participants physically or emotionally. Ethical concerns arise when techniques are used simply as gimmicks and are not designed to serve the needs of the participants. Groups can suffer from a negative image if techniques are abused, and this can overshadow the fundamental nature of a group as an arena for genuine and caring human interaction.

Questions and Activities

1. What information should you give potential clients before they enter a group, and what, if anything, should you not inform them about?
2. To ethically lead or co-lead a group, what training experiences are necessary? Should being a member in a group be a prerequisite for those who want to lead groups? What kind of group experience would you like to have as a member?
3. Imagine a setting in which a group member declines to participate in a technique or exercise you suggest. Describe how you would respond. How might this refusal have different implications depending on the stage of the group's development?
4. Describe a specific context and client, and explain how you would respond to the client's asking "What is the technique supposed to accomplish?"
5. We hold that leaders should have a theoretical rationale to support their choice of a technique. Think of some specific techniques you have used in leading a group. What was your rationale for using them?
6. Think of a situation in which a conflict is not being openly expressed within a group. What do you think you would do?
7. How do you teach your group members to confront in a constructive manner? What are the differences between confrontation and attack?
8. Do you think that psychological risks are necessarily a part of group participation? Explain. What are some specific risks related to participating in a group? Can you think of safeguards that are likely to minimize risks?
9. A client is following a technique that you have introduced and then says that she wants to stop. What would you do?
10. Under what circumstances and conditions do you believe it appropriate for a member to leave a group? Explain your position.
11. How would you explain to a group the importance of confidentiality?
12. What are some ways in which techniques might be misused that we have not talked about?
13. Describe what you regard as unethical motivations for using a technique.

14. As a leader, what advantages do you see to being self-disclosing? What are some ways in which a group leader might hide behind his or her professional role?
15. A member says to you: "I don't know you. I want you to share more of yourself personally so that I can trust you." How would you respond?
16. What kind of continuing education would you like to participate in as a way to upgrade your skills in group leading?
17. What considerations do you think are important in deciding whether a leader should touch a client?
18. What are some considerations involved in adapting techniques to the needs of culturally diverse populations? How might you modify certain techniques to fit the needs of clients who are culturally different from you?
19. You observe that several members of your group are pressuring an individual to say or do something. How do you think you might respond in this situation?
20. Explain what you believe to be the most important ethical considerations regarding group techniques. Are there any that we have failed to discuss in this chapter?

CHAPTER THREE

Techniques for Forming Groups

Introduction

Getting Groups Established

Recruiting Members

Screening and Selecting Members

Conducting a Preliminary Group Session

Preparing Parents of Minors

Setting Goals

Preparing Members to Get the Most from a Group

Preparing Leaders

Concluding Comments

Questions and Activities

Introduction

In this chapter we share some of the ways we have found for getting groups established. We describe techniques for recruiting, screening, selecting, and preparing members for effective work. Clients have a right to know the goals and procedures of a group, to be informed about their rights and responsibilities as members, and to understand the expectations leaders have for them. Participants will get the most from their group experience if leaders do some teaching about the group process at the beginning. If members are inadequately prepared, the group typically gets stuck in the initial stage because the participants are unable to work through conflicts that result from a lack of basic information. In our view, using the techniques described in this chapter is one of the best ways of ensuring that a group will move forward.

Getting Groups Established

A demanding part of conducting groups is the work you do before the first session. In an organized setting—a school, a mental health agency, a mental hospital, a clinic—you will usually need approval to organize a group. In such situations, write a proposal that clarifies your goals. If the goals are vague, neither your administrator nor the potential members will be likely to receive the idea for a group enthusiastically. With a well-thought-out proposal, you can convince potential participants or directors of the value of a group program. In addition, a carefully written proposal can prevent the confusion and misunderstandings that often derail groups.

In writing a proposal, consider these questions:

- What are your qualifications for leading the group, and how can you best present your background experience?
- What kind of group will this be? What structure will the group have?
- What will be your major functions as group leader?
- Why is a group useful for the purposes you hope to accomplish? What are the unique properties of a group that make it valuable for your particular population?
- For whom is the group designed?
- What will be the main goals of the group?
- Where will the group be held? How long will it last?
- Is your group sensitive to members with diverse backgrounds?
- Is your group easily accessible to people who are physically challenged?
- What steps will you take to ensure confidentiality?
- What topics do you expect to be explored?
- How will you deal with the potential dangers or risks of group participation?
- What evaluation procedures will you use to determine the degree to which the group has met its goals? What assessment procedures can you

devise to help members monitor the degree to which they are satisfied with their participation in the group?
- What follow-up procedures will you use to help members integrate what they have learned and evaluate this learning?

There is considerable latitude in how the ground rules for a group might be established; these rules depend on your objectives, the population, and your theoretical orientation. The examples presented next show two very different approaches to designing a group; each is based on the goals set for the group and an assessment of the needs of potential group members.

Designing a Time-Limited Group: An Illustration

I (Patrick Callanan) have offered a 16-week group in my private practice. Here is a description of the purpose and framework of this group, along with suggestions for orienting members and shaping specific group norms.

Rationale for the time limitation. This group teaches clients to become active in deciding what they want to change in their lives and provides them with tools to practice alternative behaviors. Limiting the time frame of the group frequently stimulates members to determine whether they are fully investing themselves. It is not assumed that the length of therapy is equated with its effectiveness. Some popular forms of cognitive behavioral therapy design 10- to 16-week treatment programs geared to produce change. Apart from theoretical support for shorter groups, there is another and more pragmatic reason for the reduced time. Practitioners who work with less affluent populations know the difficulty of requiring a commitment of time and money from them. It is beyond the means of many people to commit to attending a group every week for 12 months or longer. For those who are not psychologically sophisticated, a relatively long-term group may seem like a greater commitment than they are willing to make, especially when they are approaching a group experience with hesitation.

I do not mean to imply that the 16-week group is an inferior form of therapy that is geared toward the less affluent. Sixteen-week groups have many beneficial factors working in their favor. Any practitioner of group therapy has to be aware of the "cozy nest syndrome" that groups can provide. Some people succumb to it and stay endlessly in group therapy, always "working" and perhaps never changing. The 16-week group confronts members with the necessity of *doing* something in the group and also taking action outside of the group to change their lives. The members need to determine whether they are seriously committed to changing their lives.

Key features in the group's formation. This group is composed of people with a variety of personal and interpersonal problems that have prompted them to seek a therapist. The participants may have difficulty developing and maintaining close relationships. Although their problems are not severe enough to require medication or hospitalization, the members often feel "stuck" and seek some way to make changes. Here are some of the key features in designing this group:

- Attendance is stressed. If people come and go at will in a group, there is a reduction of intensity and a low level of trust. It is difficult to trust group members when they treat their commitment in a casual way. If a member expects to miss 3 or more sessions out of 16, it is usually best to ask the person to withdraw from the group.
- Members are reminded that they are in the group to find out something about themselves, not primarily to get close to people, to make friends, or to avoid loneliness.
- Clients are told that they should actively attempt to behave differently in the group than they typically do. The group provides some degree of safety for them to experiment with change.
- The group has eight members, it meets for two hours, and the members determine the agenda for the sessions as the group progresses. In addition to the weekly meetings, an extended session of six hours is scheduled at some point. This provides an opportunity to do more intensive work.

• • • • • • • • • • • • • • • • • •

A Contrasting Approach: The Long-Term Group

In contrast to time-limited groups such as the one just described by Patrick Callanan, I (Michael Russell) am especially interested in long-term groups. This format is exemplified by a psychoanalytic group I have co-led for many years. We hope to create an environment that helps members understand and modify their unconscious contributions to their present conflicts, which have their paradigms in infantile separation and individuation and oedipal rivalry. Many of the techniques for this format arise from our efforts to achieve a stable group environment and then to interpret reactions to events that threaten this stability. Contrary to our usual practice of distributing written information to members at the formation of a group, in this case we have not done so. Most of the original members of this group were themselves either therapists or persons with considerable sophistication in therapy, and we wanted to see what group norms and expectations would evolve in the absence of explicit written directives. Most of the members had previous experience in shorter intensive groups, and they typically felt they had made considerable headway with specific behavioral objectives but wanted a better grasp of persisting underlying character dynamics. For this group, rather than distribute literature, we generally hold one or more individual screening meetings, explain that we are seeking to provide a long-term group relationship in which members will be able draw from an extensive history with one another to get insight into themes developing over time.

We explain to prospective clients that they are being asked to join the group only if they are willing to commit to remaining for at least a year. We tell them that when they pay for their first meeting, they are also to put on deposit payment for their eventual last two sessions. This prepayment is required to underscore a commitment to attend for a minimum of two weeks after giving notice of their intention to terminate. Members are expected to pay for each session, even if they miss a group meeting. They are asked to call ahead to notify the group if they will need to be absent. These policies tend to accentuate the awareness that members have about the group as an important entity. The prospect of members' joining or leaving this group is inevitably an occasion for an in-depth examination of feelings such as the stability of the infantile maternal environment, which the group represents, or fears that established means of gaining "parental" attention will be disrupted.

• • • • • • • • • • • • • • • • • •

An Alternative Format: A Weeklong Residential Group

In this section we briefly describe a special type of group experience that we, along with other colleagues, conducted each summer for 25 years. (The final group met in 1997.) These residential groups were held in a mountain setting, which affords a retreat environment. Our experience in co-leading these weeklong groups provided the inspiration for us to write this book, and many of the techniques described here originated in these groups.

The philosophy underlying the activities during the weeklong residential group involves the notion that we have choices and can take steps to bring about a reconstruction of our existence. The group experience shows members that they do not have to be chained to past visions of themselves. Once early decisions and the faulty beliefs surrounding these decisions have been identified, members are able to replace self-limiting core beliefs with functional beliefs. If roles are no longer functional, the group affords an ideal place to learn more creative and productive ways of being in the world. The residential group evolves into a dynamic community that encourages interpersonal honesty and gives members permission to be who and what they are.

Much of what goes on in this personal workshop is an exploration of here-and-now reactions members have toward one another. However, the group also provides a place for members to gain a better grasp of how their family of origin is still influencing them. In many groups the members will symbolically find their siblings, mother, and father through the transference process. This is an ideal way to bring transference to life in the context of projections to certain members within the group. Again, we put the focus on the member who is having transference reactions. Rather than trying to change a parent who is not in the group, we help members become more aware of how they operate with the parent—and how they can act differently around the parent. Much of the work of a group entails learning how to be different in the symbolic family group from how they were in their own family. Indeed, the group can provide the functions of a nurturing family and enable members to experience how a family might be.

In our groups we do some work with the past if members initiate this, but we consistently attempt to help members see how what they are talking about from their past has an impact on how they think, feel, and act today. This leads to consideration of the future implications for the direction in which they are moving. Through the use of experiential techniques, members are able to identify with the life situations of one another, and the intense work of one individual frequently is a catalyst that brings others into the group in a meaningful way. This kind of intensive work is largely emotional, and it is extremely healing for members to express feelings that have welled up inside of them. The accepting atmosphere within the group provides a foundation for the participants to experience their pain and to express it. As they experience the pain associated with feelings about certain events, participants are able to release feelings and gain increased insight into some of the places where they are psychologically stuck. Once group members have given expression to feelings that have been sealed off for many years—when they have relived some of their fears and hopes—they are better able to put some meaning to these events. It is our belief that cognition is important in the healing process, but we make the assumption that people are more able to deal with their faulty beliefs once they have experienced the emotion surrounding an event.

A central dimension of the group process involves members' awareness of decisions they made about themselves in their world. Even though these early decisions were once made for the purpose of physical and psychological survival, many of these decisions may no longer serve them. The point of working with unfinished themes from childhood is to enable members to examine the degree to which their core decisions are working for them today and to begin a process of redecision. The group experience affords participants an opportunity to consider a new set of beliefs, as well as room to experiment with new ways of behaving.

For the most part, members find that this kind of intensive group experience gives them a good understanding of their significant patterns. It is too much to expect that in one week the members are able to work through many of the concerns they brought to the group, but they have a much clearer sense of work they can continue in their personal therapy. They do get a good picture of how they present themselves to others, and of how others experience and react to them. With this feedback, group members have some tools for experimenting with different ways of behaving in everyday life. Furthermore, with increased self-acceptance and self-affirmation, the participants have a basis for going beyond taking care of themselves. They are now able to genuinely be interested in others and typically demonstrate a will to make a difference in the lives of others.

Although we are aware that very few of you will design a weeklong residential group, we described this kind of group to give you a context of the environment that led to the creativity in designing the techniques you will read about—and to give you a sense of how important it is to provide a safe climate that enables members to take the risks necessary to move forward.

• • • • • • • • • • • • • • • • • •

Having described some differences between designing a time-limited group and a long-term group, and an intensive residential group experience, we now move to a discussion of specific techniques that you may find useful in forming a variety of groups, such as therapeutic groups, task groups, and psychoeducational groups. In the recruitment process for any type of group, potential clients have a right to know the goals of the group, the basic procedures to be used, what will be expected of them as participants, what they can expect of the leader, and any major risks as well as potential values of participating in the group.

Therapeutic groups. The main purposes of *therapeutic groups* are to increase people's knowledge of themselves and others, help them clarify the changes they most want to make in their lives, and give them some of the tools necessary to make these changes. By interacting with others in a trusting and accepting environment, participants are given the opportunity to experiment with novel behavior and to receive honest feedback from others concerning the effects of their behavior. As a result, individuals learn how they appear to others. The techniques we describe are primarily focused on this type of group, but many of these techniques can also be applied in other kinds of groups.

Task or work groups. Groups known as *task facilitation groups* include task forces, committees, planning groups, community organizations, discussion groups, study circles, learning groups, and other similar groups. The focus is on the application of group dynamics principles and processes to improve practice and to foster accomplishment of identified work goals.

Group workers who specialize in promoting the development and functioning of task or work groups assist participants to enhance or correct their performance. Group workers who facilitate these groups may need to be skilled in areas such as organizational assessment, training, program development, consultation, and program evaluation.

Psychoeducational groups. The *psychoeducational* group facilitator works with relatively well-functioning individuals who may have an information deficit in a certain area. The goal is to work on an array of educational deficits and psychological problems. Psychoeducational groups serve a number of purposes: presenting information about specific topics, sharing common experiences, teaching people how to solve problems, offering support, and helping people learn how to create their own support systems outside of the group setting. These groups typically focus on imparting, discussing, and integrating factual information. New information is incorporated through the use of planned skill-building exercises. Psychoeducational groups have both an educational and a therapeutic aim. Those who design and lead psychoeducational groups should have content knowledge in the topic areas in which they intend to work (such as substance abuse prevention, stress management, parent effectiveness training, assertion training, or AIDS).

Regardless of the type of group you are leading, some common factors generally need to be addressed in designing the group: leaders need to be clear about what they most hope to accomplish; leaders have the task of developing a proposal to market the group; and leaders need to think about the best ways to announce the group, screen potential candidates, and select and orient the members. Although therapeutic groups differ from both task facilitation groups and psychoeducational groups, many common principles can be applied to forming any group.

In the remaining sections we consider strategies for recruiting, screening, selecting, and preparing members for a group. Our focus is on the importance of the preliminary group session for orientation purposes and on techniques for assisting members in defining and clarifying their personal goals. We also list guidelines and suggestions for members to derive the maximum benefit from a group.

Recruiting Members

Personal contact is the best way to recruit potential candidates for a group, because members are committing themselves to working with a specific person. In addition, through personal contact the leader can demonstrate that the group has potential value for a person.

Rather than simply relying on flyers, leaders can contact people who might direct clients to them: colleagues, directors of clinics, teachers and professors, physicians, ministers, school counselors, psychologists, and social workers. It is a group leader's responsibility to become familiar with the resources in the community and to educate referral sources. Indeed, this is probably the best method of recruiting potential group members.

Screening and Selecting Members

With respect to both therapeutic groups and psychoeducational groups, the next step is to determine who might profit from the group and who (if anyone) should be excluded. One technique for making these decisions is to meet privately with every person who wishes to join the group. In such a meeting the leader can get a sense of the appropriateness of including particular candidates and can give them a chance to determine whether they want to be involved. Leaders need to keep in mind that all groups are not appropriate for all people. Indeed, for some, group participation can be damaging or at least counterproductive to their growth. The question of the appropriateness of including a member is directly related to the purpose and goals of the group. Let's assume that a candidate for a group, Wilma, meets with the therapist for a half-hour individual screening session. She can also ask questions of the leader to help her determine if she wants to be in this group. Ideally, the interview will be a two-way exchange in which a mutual decision is made. The leader can ask questions such as the following of Wilma to get a sense of her readiness for the group:

- Why do you want to join the group?
- Have you participated in a group or in individual therapy before? What was that experience like for you?
- Do you understand the purposes and nature of this group?
- Do you have any fears about joining this group?
- How ready are you to take a critical look at your life or address a particular problem you are facing?
- What are some specific personal concerns that you'd most like to explore?
- What would you most hope to get from this group?
- What do you want to know about me?

This individual contact between the prospective member and the leader can be extremely useful as a way to begin to establish trust, for it can allay fears and provide the foundation for future work. Of course, orientation interviews are time consuming and may not always be feasible, but they are worth the time that they take. Even a brief contact significantly reduces risk and contributes to the overall quality of the group. For example, in a psychoeducational group, some people may be expecting a personal experience aimed at changing aspects of their personality. They may be seeking a therapy group, which would not be congruent with the goals and purposes of a psychoeducational group. This initial contact provides prospective members with some idea of what to expect, and thus they are more likely to come prepared to work if they decide to join the group.

Sometimes it is impossible to individually screen prospective members. For instance, you may work in a residential facility where groups are formed on the basis of people who live on the same ward. When screening is not possible, it is important to devise some alternative strategy. At least you can meet with individuals on the ward before they are placed in your group and orient them to the process. If time constraints make it impractical for you to screen each member individually, you can experiment with group interviews.

Leaders have a responsibility to make a determination as to whether or not a prospective member is suitable for a given group, which is for the protection of the prospective member and the group itself. They need to inform prospective members that a particular group could be more harmful than helpful to them. If leaders deem that members are not appropriate for a group, they have a responsibility to give reasons for this decision and to make an appropriate referral. For example, a leader might say something like this to a member who will not be accepted into a group: "During the initial screening interview, you mentioned that you are taking psychotropic medication. At this time it would not be in your best interests to put you into a group where intense emotions are likely to be expressed. I would recommend that you pursue some individual therapy, for which I can make some referrals. At a future date, should you reapply, I would be happy to reconsider." We wish to add that it is not the existence of the medication that the person is taking but rather his or her emotional stability that is key in making this decision.

Conducting a Preliminary Group Session

In addition to an individual meeting, we also recommend a preliminary group session with the potential members. This is true for both therapeutic groups and psychoeducational groups. The primary purpose of this meeting is for the leader to outline the aims of the group in detail and to clarify what the participants will be doing. It gives participants an opportunity to meet one another and to get additional data for making their decision about committing themselves to the group. A preliminary session is an excellent time to introduce the necessities for informed consent.

Such a meeting has the following specific purposes: getting acquainted; clarifying personal goals and group goals; learning about the procedures to be used in the group; learning how the group will function and how to get the most from the experience; discussing the possible dangers or risks involved in participating in the group and ways of minimizing these risks; discussing the essential requirement of confidentiality and any other necessary ground rules; exploring with members their fears, expectations, hopes, and ambivalent feelings; and answering their questions. During this preliminary group meeting, members sometimes have few questions, and in those cases we tend to raise questions that we know are frequently on the minds of people who are about to enter a group. Here are some examples of questions that members have brought to a preliminary session:

- Will I be pressured to say more than I want?
- Can I expect there to be opportunities to work on exploring and solving particular problems in my life?
- Will this group teach me new information and equip me with skills to better cope with a range of everyday problems?
- Is everything that we say confidential?
- If I get scared, is it acceptable to leave a session?
- How much will you leaders be sharing with us personally? Will you also be members?
- What kind of techniques will you use?
- What are some problems that people typically talk about? Is there anything we shouldn't talk about?
- How will I know if I am fitting in this group?
- Do I need to attend every session?

Some of these questions may be interesting to explore in depth later, but we answer them in a straightforward manner at this time. At the end of the first session, individuals can be asked to think about whether they still want to join the group. A leader who has reservations about admitting a member can arrange for another interview to explore these reservations.

Let's look at specific matters that need to be openly explored at these initial meetings for both therapeutic and psychoeducational groups. One is confidentiality. Members will not feel free to explore issues in a meaningful way if they don't have the assurance that what they say will be held in confidence by both the leaders and the other members. Members need to be reminded emphatically about how easily they may unintentionally breach the confidences of other members by talking about specifics brought up in the group. And leaders must state directly and openly any limitations of confidentiality. They should inform members of the circumstances under which they will have to divulge material that is brought up in the group. It is a good idea to have a written statement clarifying the dimensions of confidentiality, which members sign indicating their understanding and agreement of the ramifications of confidentiality. Such a statement is especially important in a mandatory group in a detention facility. For example, if a group leader must report on the clients' progress, he or she should clearly point out this requirement and make it a topic for discussion. Other limitations of confidentiality include the legal requirement to report cases of suspected child abuse or incest or to report situations involving potential harm to the client or others.

Some basic matters that might be mentioned at the preliminary session include policies on eating during group meetings, coming to the group on time, missing group sessions, socializing outside the group and other subgrouping matters, and having sessions recorded.

For any kind of group, the best technique is for the leader to simply state some essential procedures and policies and discuss them in the group. In addition, the leader can distribute two copies of a list of the important group procedures and policies to each member. Members can sign both copies, keeping one and giving the other to the group leader. Leaders who use this technique as a way of clarifying and focusing on procedures and policies should go over the policies with the members and express the reasons for establishing them. Following is a typical list of ground rules for a group.

Ground Rules for Groups

1. Members are not to use drugs or alcohol during a session and are not to come to a session under the influence of any chemical agents.
2. Members are expected to be present at all the group meetings because their absence affects the entire group.
3. Members must avoid sexual involvement with others in the group during its duration.
4. Members are not to use physical violence in group sessions, nor are they to be verbally abusive to others in the group.
5. Members will be given a summary of their rights and responsibilities so that they know what is expected of them before they join the group.

6. Members must keep confidential what other members do and say within the group.
7. Members are informed about the limits of confidentiality.

• • • • • • • • • • • • • • • • • •

Because of time constraints, a preliminary session may not be feasible in all cases, even though it is highly recommended. As a substitute, group leaders can integrate many of the ideas we cover here in the first session. The initial group meeting can then be an orientation session during which members decide whether the group is appropriate for them. Even if your group meets for as few as six sessions, some type of preliminary orientation session would be very helpful. We suggest adding one session for this preliminary preparation of members.

Preparing Parents of Minors

In planning a group composed of children or adolescents, it is generally wise to contact the parents or legal guardians of the potential members and secure their written permission before allowing the members to enroll in the group. However, the practice of informed consent and of getting parental permission for counseling services varies from school to school and from state to state. Be sure you understand the requirements where your groups are held.

An additional technique is to invite parents and their children to a meeting with you to present the need for such a group and to discuss their questions or concerns. Sending letters to parents and holding a meeting with them and their children can prevent many problems from developing later. If parents are not informed or their cooperation is not enlisted, conflicts may result, which could be harmful to the children. For example, some parents may think that family matters will be publicly aired or that their children will be brainwashed. Your presentation can put to rest some of the false notions that parents may have about the group. As laws and policies vary from state to state, and agency to agency, we seek to inform parents about how much we will or will not disclose to them pertaining to their children.

Setting Goals

Members and leaders need to set goals for themselves, both at the start of a group and at the start of each session, for maximum learning to occur. Members can begin to set these goals at the screening interview and also at the preliminary session. We describe in this section some techniques the leader may want to use in this process. We hope that you will not consider the activities we describe as school assignments but as focusing methods. These are merely suggestions to choose from, and you would not want to use all these techniques in one group.

The kind of preparation we discuss here can be used in any group, but it is particularly useful in giving direction to groups, such as those for children, that need a significant degree of structure to function effectively. Maintain a balance between too much structure and not enough. Too much structure may squelch the creativity and self-direction of group members, and not enough preparation may cause a group to flounder needlessly because of a lack of focus. Another factor to consider in deciding on the degree of structure is the leader's theoretical orientation, experience, training, and personal characteristics. Some leaders work better with more structure, some with less.

Psychoeducational groups often focus on a particular theme. A few examples of psychoeducational groups that are structured with topics around a central theme include groups for managing stress, dealing with life transitions, acquiring coping skills, learning ways to enhance interpersonal functioning, dealing with body image, learning assertiveness, and parent education. Structured groups with an educational focus are increasingly common in agencies, schools, and college counseling centers. Although the specific topic varies according to the interests of the leader and the population of the group, such groups share the aim of providing members with increased awareness of some life problem and the tools to better cope with it.

At the beginning of these structured groups, it is common to ask members to complete a questionnaire on how well they are coping with the area of concern. Such groups make use of structured exercises, readings, homework assignments, and contracts. When the group comes to an end, another questionnaire is often used to assess members' progress.

The group leader will have general goals in mind for the group, and in psychoeducational groups these goals may be geared toward behavior change. However, unless the group leader pays attention to creating a safe atmosphere that will enable participants to address topics in a personal way, these goals are not likely to be accomplished. In counseling and therapy groups, process goals may be the focus, such as learning appropriate self-disclosure, being willing to share feelings, being willing to talk in a personal way, staying in the here-and-now, expressing reactions to what is going on in the group, learning how to confront with care and respect, and learning how to give others feedback. If members know these goals from the start, they have a clear idea of what is expected of them and also how they might get the most from the group for themselves.

In addition, members of any kind of group need to clarify what they want from the group. Their thinking on this matter is often fuzzy and global. They hope to get in touch with their feelings, they would like to communicate better, they hope to solve a problem, or they want to work on understanding themselves. These vague goals are hard to work on in a group. Helping members translate general goals into specific ones is the first step in preparation. Thus, if a member says, "I want to learn how to express my feelings," the leader might ask: "What particular feeling do you have the most trouble expressing? In what situations do you find it most difficult to express this feeling? What's it like for you to be this way? How would you like to be different?"

Asking members to tell one another of their specific goals is one way to get them to think about their reasons for being in the group. Having them write down these goals is valuable. One technique that some of our student leaders have used in their groups is to ask their members at the first session to write a letter to themselves, which will be opened at the last meeting. The participants are asked to write a paragraph on what they would most like to say they had gotten out of the group experience. At the final session, the members unseal their letters and decide whether to share with others what they wrote to themselves. A variation is to ask people to write down at an early session what they hope to have done, or how they hope to have changed in six months or a year. They give these statements to the leader in sealed envelopes, and the leader returns them unopened at the end of the time period. Not only do such exercises challenge members to look at what they want for themselves, but they are also a device for accountability. These letter techniques can be useful in helping members focus on what they want from a group experience as well as what they would like to do in applying this experience to their everyday lives.

Preparing contracts. A full contract is an extension of the letter-writing techniques. In designing contracts, members write out the specific behaviors or attitudes they want to change and what they are willing to do inside and outside the group to make these changes. The contract method can be useful for counseling groups, therapy groups, and psychoeducational groups. Members can compose these contracts at home after the first session, bring them back to the group at the second meeting, and discuss them in the group. The leader and other members can offer their perceptions of how realistic the person's goals are and can offer other ways to meet the objectives. Here are some guidelines to assist in designing effective contracts:

- Keep the language concise and specific.
- State goals in behavioral terms.
- Strive for realistic and attainable goals.
- Identify short- and long-term goals.
- Relate personal goals to the general goals and purpose of the group.

Contracts should not be compared to legal documents; rather, they provide a strategy for helping members be specific about those thoughts, feelings, and actions they would like to change. The contract can spell out how they intend to make the change, a schedule for doing so, and possible strategies for coping with setbacks to their plans.

Reading. Reading can be a great asset to the members of both psychoeducational groups and therapeutic groups. By doing some reading before the group begins, participants solidify their commitment and focus. Reading can assist them in reflecting on their lives and on what they want to change. For example, a psychoeducational group might be structured to teach participants how to be assertive in various situations and to assist members in acquiring skills in assertive behavior. As a route to best learning this knowledge and gaining these skills, the members can read books dealing with assertiveness training.

Reading can be used as a focusing technique in other ways. You may be aware of a specific theme that a particular member of the group plans to explore and be able to recommend a book that helps the member focus on that topic. You may also ask members to select from among the many self-help paperbacks some that they expect might be useful for them. Or you may give them a bibliography about groups or about probable group topics and urge them to select those that they think might be especially meaningful at this point in their lives. You may also encourage group participants to reread a book that has had an impact on them or to reread their favorite childhood fairy tale and reflect on whether it symbolized any struggles they faced. Reading can prime people to think about issues in their lives that they would like to bring to a group. It is also a way of getting people to continue working between sessions.

Writing journals. Writing can be used in several ways as an adjunct to preparation for either a psychoeducational group or therapeutic group or for a specific group meeting. Members can spend 10 minutes each day recording in a journal certain feelings, situations, behaviors, and ideas for courses of action. For example, clients who are working at being assertive can make journal entries about the inner dialogue they have before deciding to express an idea, about times they did express an opinion (how they felt, how others reacted to them), about times they sat quietly thinking they had nothing valuable to offer (and how they felt then), and about how to change these patterns.

Members can also review certain periods of time in their lives and write about them. For example, they can get out pictures of their childhood years and other reminders of this period and then freely write in a journal whatever comes to mind. Writing in a free-flowing style without censoring can be of great help in getting a focus on feelings.

One of our colleagues has conducted a psychoeducational group for men in a community agency for more than 10 years. The group is topically oriented, educationally and therapeutically focused, and combines a variety of techniques. At an early group session the men are invited to explore gender-related issues such as what it means to be a man, the messages they received in growing up, and how these messages affect them today. Later sessions are structured around relationships with parents, relationships with significant others, developing and maintaining friendships, relationships with children, work, sexuality, and other topics that the men initiate for discussion. Members are generally given some kind of reading material prior to each session. They are also encouraged to keep a journal and write about their thoughts and feelings pertaining to the topics for each session. They are asked to write about their reactions to each of the group meetings, which gives them an opportunity to reflect on each session during the week.

For many types of groups, the members can bring the journals to the group and share a particular experience they had that resulted in problems for them. They can then explore with the group how they might have handled the situation differently. In general, however, these journals are for the benefit of the members, to help them focus themselves for a session. The members themselves can decide what they do with the material they write.

Another way to use journals is as a preparation for encountering others in everyday life. For instance, Jenny is having a great deal of difficulty talking with her husband. She's angry with him much of the time over many of the things he does and does not do. But she sits on this anger, and she feels sad that they don't take time for each other. Jenny typically doesn't express her sadness to him, nor does she let him know of her resentment toward him for not being involved in their children's lives. To deal with this problem, she can write her husband a detailed and uncensored letter pointing out all the ways in which she feels angry, hurt, sad, and disappointed and expressing how she would like their life to be different. It is not necessary that she show this letter to her husband. The letter writing is a way for her to clarify what she does feel and to prepare herself to work in the group. This work can then help her to be clear about what she wants to say to her husband as well as how she wants to say it. This process works in the following way: Jenny can say aloud some of what she wrote to a member in the group who role-plays her husband. Others can then express how they experience her and the impact she has on them. Aided by such feedback, she may be able to hit on a constructive way of expressing her feelings to her husband in real life.

Still another technique is for members to spontaneously enter in their journals their reactions to themselves in the group:

- What is it like to be in this group?
- How do I see people in the group? How do I see myself in it?
- How do I sabotage myself so that I don't get what I might from this group? How can I challenge myself when I become aware of defeating myself?
- What are some ways in which I avoid?

If people write down their reactions in this way, they are likely to verbalize them in the group. For instance, if members fear opening up lest others see them as being stupid, this fear prevents them from sharing their concerns. If they write about this fear and then bring it up for consideration in the group, they lessen their chances of being stopped by the fear.

Another useful technique is for people to write down their reactions to each session. A brief review of the session provides them with a running account of their experiences in the group. As the group is coming to an end, these notes can be useful in recalling and understanding specific events.

Writing can be useful as the group progresses as well as during the early stage. At the midpoint of a group, people can take time during the week to write down how they feel about the group at this point, how they view their participation in it so far, what they are doing outside the group to attain their goals, and how they would feel if the group ended right now. By discussing these statements in the group, participants are challenged to reevaluate their level of commitment and are often motivated to increase their participation in the group.

Using structured questionnaires. A sentence-completion questionnaire that includes the following statements might be administered to many different kinds of groups in an early session:

- What I most want from this group is _______.
- The one thing I'd most want to be able to say at our final meeting is _______.
- Thinking about being in this group for the next 20 weeks, I _______.
- A fear I have about being a group member is _______.
- One personal concern I would hope to bring up is _______.
- I often feel _______.
- The one aspect I'd most like to change about myself is _______.
- Something I particularly like about myself is _______.

This is a focusing device, and it can be followed with a discussion of whatever it brings out in the members.

A problem checklist is another valuable tool for helping members decide how they want to use the group time. For an adolescent group, for example, develop a list of problems teenagers typically face and ask members to write down the degree to which each problem applies to them (anonymously if they wish). The following inventory is an illustration.

Problem Checklist for an Adolescent Group

Directions: Rate each of the following problems as they apply to you at this time, and indicate the degree to which you'd like help from the group with them using this scale:

1 = This is a major problem for me, one I hope will be a topic for exploration in the group.
2 = This is a problem for me at times, and I could profit from an open discussion of the matter in this group.
3 = This is not a concern of mine, and I don't feel a need to explore the topic in the group.

_____ 1. Feeling accepted by my peer group
_____ 2. Learning how to trust others
_____ 3. Getting along with my parents (brothers, sisters)

_____ 4. Getting a clear sense of what I value
_____ 5. Being fearful of relating to the same sex
_____ 6. Being fearful of relating to the opposite sex
_____ 7. Dealing with sexual feelings, actions, and standards of behavior
_____ 8. Being so concerned about doing what is expected of me that I don't live by my own standards
_____ 9. Worrying about my future
_____ 10. Wondering whether I will get into college
_____ 11. Trying to decide on a career

Additional problems I'd like to pursue:

____

____

• • • • • • • • • • • • • • • • • •

A questionnaire does not have to be this elaborate. In an adolescent group, for example, one could simply ask: "What problems would your parents like you to discuss in this group, and what would you like to say about these problems? What issues might your peers suggest to you for exploration in this group?"

Constructing a critical turning points chart. Another technique to prepare members for productive work is asking them to draw a road map of their lives and include some of the following points of interest: key turning points, major crises, big decisions, new opportunities, major accomplishments, severe failures, important people, and major disappointments. Members can then work in pairs, selecting whatever they would like to share from their charts. Or they can talk about critical turning points in their lives with the entire group. In addition to or in place of a chart, clients can draw a sketch divided into three parts: "My Past/My Present/My Future." Much of their drawing may be symbolic. Again, they can share what parts of their sketch mean to them in small groups or in the group as a whole.

Writing an autobiography. Another technique for getting members focused is to ask them to write autobiographies in which they present their current subjective views of various points in their lives: childhood, adolescence, early adulthood. They can be encouraged to stress significant events, persistent emotions, dreams, relationships with others, and parallels in their lives at present. They might pay particular attention to those events that evoked intense emotions, because these may contain clues to work they decide to pursue in the group. It helps to ask members not to write merely factual accounts of their lives but, instead, to focus on the personal meaning that certain events had for them. For example, a male member may write about ways in which his parents' divorce affected him during his adolescence.

He may talk about feeling guilty and responsible for the breakup of his parents. Another member, a young woman, may write about how incest during her adolescence continues to influence her as an adult. Another member may talk about a midlife career change that she made and the flak that she received from her family. She could write about how the negative reactions from her children and husband are still affecting her. The useful feature of writing autobiographies is that core material can be brought into group sessions for further exploration.

Using fantasy. An open-structured or nondirective fantasy technique can be useful in the early stages of a group for individual focusing, for providing data, and for getting group members acquainted with one another. One such exercise, which can be done either in writing or orally, goes like this: "Imagine that you are a book. What's a good title for you that captures something of what you are all about? What's your style, your tone? What are your chapter headings? How about your cover and your preface—will people be enticed to read you? Are you going to deliver what you advertise? Which chapters of you were the hardest to write? Which chapters would you want to have deleted? After people have read through you, cover to cover, what do you suppose they will think?"

The same device can be used during the ending stages of a group when members are being asked to consolidate their group experience: "Thinking back to the book you imagined yourself to be at the beginning of this group, do you want now to have a different title? What other changes and revisions would you like to make, from beginning to end?"

Preparing Members to Get the Most from a Group

Encouraging members to prepare themselves to actively participate in each group session is critical for both psychoeducational and therapeutic groups. At the initial session you can discuss with members some guidelines for involving themselves in the group and applying what they learn to their daily lives. To gain the most from a variety of different groups, participants need to be oriented and prepared. Of course, there is a danger in overpreparing members. By spending too much time teaching them what to look for and how to act, you run the risk of doing too much of the work that the group ultimately needs to do for itself. Even though not every possibility needs to be covered, some preparation at the outset can create a climate conducive to productive work as the group moves into its advanced stages.

In many ways, the norms that govern group behavior are foreign to the expected behavior in daily living. Group members are expected to express feelings, to ask directly for what they want, to take time for themselves, to allow themselves to be vulnerable, to tell others how they affect them, to deal with conflict, and to make decisions for themselves. Members can also be expected to assess their belief systems and how their thinking is influencing what they are doing and how they are feeling. Many of these behavioral standards are contrary to the process of socialization that most perienced. Members need to acquire a mind-set for how to a pate in an interpersonal group. All this preparation doesn't h pleted at the initial session, and much of it needs to be re discussed during the first few meetings.

The best way to distribute this information is to write it down and give it to members at the screening interview, the preliminary session, or the first group session. The following guidelines are designed for growth groups for relatively well-functioning adults, but some of these guidelines can be applied to psychoeducational groups too. The list can be shortened or modified depending on the specific population and the particular type of group.

Guidelines and Suggestions for Group Members

1. *Have a focus.* Commit yourself to getting something from this group by focusing on what you hope to accomplish. In clarifying your goals, review specific issues you want to explore, specific changes you want to make, and actions you are willing to take to make these changes. Before each group session, take time to clarify what you would like to bring up during that meeting, and write these issues down if that is helpful to you.

2. *Be flexible.* Although it helps to approach a group session with some idea of what you want to explore, don't be so committed to your agenda that you cannot work with what comes up spontaneously within the group. Be open to pursuing alternative paths if you are affected by others in your group.

3. *Don't wait to work.* It is easy to let a group session go by without getting around to what you hope to do or say. The longer you wait to involve yourself, the harder it will become. Therefore, challenge yourself to have something to say at the beginning of each group, even if it's a brief statement of what it was like for you to come to the group that day.

4. *Be "greedy."* The success of a group depends on your being eager to do your own work. This doesn't mean that you should monopolize time or be insensitive to the difficulty others may have in getting into the spotlight. But if you constantly wait until it's your "turn" or try to monitor how much of the group's time should be allotted to you, you will inhibit the spontaneity and enthusiasm that can make a group exciting and productive. If each member takes responsibility for pursuing his or her own work, everyone should have enough opportunity to speak.

5. *Pay attention to feelings.* Intellectual discussions are great, but an experiential group is also about your feelings and convictions, not just your thinking. If you do nothing but expound your theories and opinions, you will not explore your life on an emotional level. As a guideline, if your sentences can just as well start "My opinion is that _______," you probably are not working much on a feeling level, and you are not taking full advantage of the unique opportunity for doing so that an experiential group provides. You don't need to work hard to generate feelings, but be open to letting

yourself experience them as you are in a session and as you are present for others. Also, if you are talking about a topic in the group, find some way to show how this matter is connected with you personally. Avoid abstract discussions of topics that have no personal relevance.

6. *Express yourself.* Most of us are in the habit of censoring our expression of thoughts and feelings. We are afraid of being inappropriate or, often, afraid that we will simply magnify and entrench the feelings and convictions we have if we voice them. These fears are not unfounded, but we have far more reason to be concerned about what we do to ourselves when we don't verbalize than when we do. And experientially there is a world of difference between thinking something through in our minds and saying it out loud. A group is an ideal place to find out what would happen if we expressed what we felt, which can be a powerful and positive experience. If you have feelings that relate to the group, be willing to express them. For example, if you are aware of feeling bored, announce that you feel this way, and be willing to take responsibility for your own boredom. Keeping these sorts of things to yourself is a sure way to dam up the flow of a group.

7. *Be an active participant.* You will help yourself most if you take an active role in the group. Members who are silent observers are not likely to benefit as much from their participation in the group, and others may believe their silence means they are being judgmental. Although members who tend to be quiet may be learning vicariously, they deprive others of the opportunity to learn from them. Realize that others will not know you if you remain silent on issues that are important to you. At least let people know what it is like for you to be in a particular group session. Even if you did not do any focused work yourself during the session, you are likely to have had reactions to what went on with others. Let them know how their work affected you.

8. *Experiment.* Look at the group as a place in which you are safer and freer than usual to express yourself in different ways and to try out different sides of yourself. Having done so, you can then seek ways of carrying these new behaviors into your outside life. In between group meetings, think of specific ways in which you can practice and experiment with the behaviors you are acquiring in your group. Then, report to the group how you are letting yourself behave differently outside.

9. *Be willing to explore.* Groups are built on the assumption that no matter how well your life may be going now, it can be enriched by the opportunity to explore your feelings, values, beliefs, attitudes, and thoughts and to consider changes you may want to make. If you believe such exploration is appropriate only for people with severe emotional problems, you are shortchanging yourself and the other participants. Even though you do not have any pressing crisis in your life, assume that the issues that come up for you are worth exploring.

10. *Don't expect change to be instantaneous.* If you do seek to change some features of your life, remember that such changes do not usually happen all at once or without some backsliding. Don't be overly critical of yourself if you

experience setbacks. Realize that it will take time to change longstanding patterns and that there may be a tendency to revert to familiar ways when you are faced with stressful situations. Give yourself credit for what you are willing to try and for subtle changes you can see yourself making.

11. *Don't expect others to appreciate your changes.* Some people in your life may have an investment in keeping you the way you are now. You may find less support for your struggles outside the group than within it. Use the group to explore ways to handle the resistance you encounter outside. It is a good idea to remind yourself that you are in this group primarily to make the changes that you want in yourself, not to change someone else. It may happen that you come to understand others more fully or that others in your life change in response to your being different, but don't focus on them primarily.

12. *Don't expect to be fully understood within the group.* Groups heighten a sense of intimacy and provide an opportunity for being understood by others in ways we don't always experience in our daily lives. Even in groups, however, it is unlikely that you will be fully understood. Members will see certain dimensions of you but will not have a good idea of what you are like otherwise. If you are working mainly on conflicts or emotional vulnerability, the group will see this side of you. You can waste your time and everyone else's if you feel you must constantly qualify and footnote everything you express. A concern that everyone get the full picture—which probably is impossible anyway—will just distract you from achieving your goals in the group. For example, if you choose to explore some feelings you have about a relationship you are in and think you must explain those feelings by giving a full and "objective" account of the relationship, you will be talking forever. Better to resign yourself in advance to the idea that others won't and can't have the full picture.

13. *Don't expect to fully understand others in the group.* You do a disservice to others in the group if you suppose that you have them all figured out. Like you, they are presumably working on expressing a side of themselves that they do not usually have an opportunity to express. If you let yourself think that that's the whole picture, you are forgetting how complex people are.

14. *Stick with one feeling at a time.* You will have much more opportunity to learn new behavior if you immediately express yourself rather than trying to put things into perspective. A good way to keep yourself from facing anything is to censor your expression of one sort of feeling because you are in a hurry to express a contrary feeling. You may have mixed emotions about an issue, but if you want to fully face that issue, try to stick with those feelings one at a time.

15. *Avoid advising, interpreting, and questioning.* As you listen to others in the group, you will often be tempted to offer advice. People can easily be inundated by well-meant advice. They are likely to withdraw, and you are likely to forget that you are in the group to express yourself. Your contribution will be much better received if it consists not of giving advice but of expressing feelings and experiences of your own that the person stimulated. Similarly, when everyone starts taking on the role of the group leader in providing

interpretations, the person speaking is likely to feel that he or she is the only one working and become defensive. People also tend to be defensive when faced with an onslaught of questions. Questions can be asked in ways that open people up rather than closing them down. If you are inclined to ask a question, experiment with prefacing your question with a declaration of why you have an interest in hearing someone's answer. Let others know of your personal investment in your questions. You will carry your work further if you tell them your personal reactions to the issue rather than questioning them about theirs. Questions that come from genuine concern mean more than those that spring from mere curiosity.

16. *Don't "gossip."* Gossiping is talking about someone in the third person. If the person is not in the room, your group leader may encourage you to pretend that the person you want to talk about is in the room and have you speak directly to this person. Although this exercise may seem artificial at times, it usually leads to a powerful expression of feelings or thoughts. If you doubt this result, watch how the exercise works with others in your group. Or think of someone toward whom you feel anger and see whether you can experience the difference by first saying aloud "I'm angry with him because _______" and then saying "I'm angry with you because_______."

17. *Don't be too quick to comfort.* If you rush in to support or comfort fellow members who are expressing pain, you may not be respecting their ability and desire to fully express what they want to say. You probably know from your own experience how good it can feel to get something out instead of having it cut off by someone's ill-timed helpfulness. People grow from living through their pain, so let them do it. Certainly, interactions in a group leave plenty of room for words and gestures of comfort or consolation, but wait until people have gotten through their pain.

18. *Give feedback.* When people express something that touches you, let them know by sharing your own feelings and reactions. Even if your feedback is not easy to express and may be difficult to listen to, it can be useful if it is delivered in a caring and respectful manner. In the long run, your willingness to directly and honestly confront another member with your reactions enhances the level of trust within the group and leads you to greater honesty in your daily life. When providing others with feedback, steer clear of telling them what they should do or how they are. Avoid giving quick reassurance or offering them pat solutions for their problems. Rather than telling them how to solve their problems, tell them about your own struggle with your own problems. Emphasize feedback that will give others a dearer sense of how their behavior affects you personally. Avoid judging people, but do let them know what specific behaviors of theirs might be getting in your way in dealing with them. Also, let them know of behaviors that might bring you closer to them.

19. *Be open to feedback.* When others give you feedback about their reactions to your work, remember that, like you, they are there to try out new ways of expressing themselves directly. It is easy to accept their feedback as gospel or to be too quick to reject their insights by rebutting them or ex-

plaining away what they say. The most constructive approach is usually to listen and to think their reactions over until you get a grasp on what parts of it fit.

20. *Avoid storytelling.* If you go on at length to provide others with information about you, you wind up distracting yourself and everyone else. Avoid narratives of your history. Express what is present, or express what is past if you are struggling with this past event.

21. *Exaggerate.* You can sometimes worry too much about whether you are genuine when you focus on a feeling you have. Rather than wondering whether you are exaggerating your emotions, give yourself permission to nurture them a bit and discover where they lead. Of course, you won't want to fake it, but you may get in touch with something genuine by throwing yourself into what you feel.

22. *Avoid sarcasm.* A main goal of participants in an experiential group is to learn to express feelings, including anger, in a direct manner. If you feel angry, say so directly. Do not use pot shots and sarcasm, which people often don't know how to interpret. If you are hostile, which is indirect anger, not only does this negatively affect others around you but it also builds up inside of you. If you learn to express even minor irritations, there is a reduced risk that you will store up negative reactions that are unexpressed, which eventually lead to hostility and are expressed through sarcasm.

23. *Include group leaders in your reactions.* It is normal for members to react to group leaders with feelings borrowed from the past, from fantasy, and from reality. You can turn this reaction to advantage by making it a special point to explore and express your feelings about your group leaders. Let them know how what they are saying and doing affects you.

24. *Beware of labels.* Watch out for the generalizations, summary statements, and labels you use to describe yourself. For example, you may define yourself as a "loner" and an "outsider," and you may communicate through your behavior that you want people to stay away. Such behavior and self-imposed labels invite others to treat you as an outsider and insist on pigeonholing you for the duration of the group. Be ready to challenge others if you think they are reducing you to one dimension. Don't assume that labels tell you all there is to know about you or someone else.

25. *Make friends with your defenses.* Your defenses have helped you get where you are today. But they may need modification if you are to make significant changes. Come to respect your defenses by understanding the purpose they serve. You probably already have some idea of how you might sabotage your own work in a group by rationalizing, withdrawing, denying, or turning a specific criticism into a global "I'm no good." When you become aware of your typical patterns of avoidance, challenge these defenses and try to substitute direct and effective behavior.

26. *Decide for yourself how much to disclose.* To find out about yourself, you need to take some risks by saying more than you are comfortable saying. However, pushing yourself should be distinguished from disclosing things about yourself simply because others seem to expect or need it. If you find

that it is difficult for you to share yourself personally in your group, begin by letting others know what makes it hard for you to let yourself be known. Group is a good place to challenge your own boundaries—but it is also a good place to respect them.

27. *Carry your work outside the group.* You will be finding new ways of expressing yourself within the group. Try these behaviors out in your everyday life with due respect for timing and with caution. But don't burden yourself with the expectation that you should express everything that you say in a group situation to a significant person in your life on the outside. For instance, you may role-play with your "father" in a group and discharge feelings of hurt and anger that you have never shared with him. If you value improving your relationship with him, it may not be wise to say everything that you released and worked through in a symbolic way in therapy. Instead, decide what you'd most want to say to him, including what you'd like to tell him about yourself. Be willing to set action-oriented homework assignments for yourself and make a commitment to yourself and your group to follow through with your plans. If you become aware that you want a closer relationship and would like to spend more time with your father, challenge yourself to carry out behavioral assignments that will help you get what you say you want. Remember, change requires that you work and practice outside of the group.

28. *Don't be stopped by setbacks.* You may have a specific vision of how you'd like to behave differently. In spite of formulating specific plans and making a commitment to accomplish your plans, however, you will have relapses at times. Instead of getting discouraged and convincing yourself that you'll never change, be patient with temporary regressions. Realize that you have spent years developing your present patterns. When you are under pressure, you may revert to these old and familiar styles, even though they may not serve you well any longer. Making the changes that you want is often a slow and tedious process.

29. *Express your feelings.* Some feelings are easier to express than others. Groups generally focus on those feelings that are causing members some difficulty. Because we usually don't get a chance to explore ways in which our feelings affect us, try to push yourself to talk about those feelings that you frequently try to deny. But you needn't conclude that there is an unspoken rule in the group that limits you to speaking only of problems and conflicts. Share your joys too!

30. *Think about your thinking.* Learn to monitor your self-talk. Identify those beliefs that work against you. For example, if you tell yourself that other members could not possibly like you or want a friendship with you once they really got to know you, reflect on how you can easily be setting yourself up for defeat. You may be creating a host of self-fulfilling prophecies that keep you from feeling and acting the way you'd like. Once you have identified some patterns of negative thinking, bring them to a session, and begin to challenge them. You can learn how to argue with those voices in your head that keep you from becoming the person you want to be.

31. *Take responsibility for what you accomplish.* The leaders and members of your group will no doubt be interested in drawing you out, but remember that in the last analysis what you accomplish in the group is up to you. Don't wait for others to call on you. Learn to ask for what you want. You will determine what and how much you get.

32. *Be familiar with your culture.* Recognize that your cultural background does influence who you are. Discover the ways in which you continue to be affected by your cultural environment. Although you can appreciate values that you have gotten from your culture, be open to questioning the degree to which you might want to modify some of them. You can ask yourself whether certain ways of living are still in your best interest. If you decide that some behaviors are no longer effective, use the group to think of ways to make the changes you desire.

33. *Develop a reading program.* Reading can be therapeutic and can also provide you with material to bring up in your therapy. Select books that will help you put your life experiences in a new perspective or books that can teach you new patterns of thinking and behaving.

34. *Write in your journal.* If you hope to rely on memory alone to sort through all that you experience in your group, you'll probably find that much of what you did and observed will be lost. Even brief entries in a journal can be useful in helping you monitor yourself to keep track of how well you are attaining your goals.

35. *Respect confidentiality.* Keep in mind how easy it might be to inadvertently betray the confidences of others. Make it a practice not to talk about what others are doing in your group or what they are experiencing. If you choose to talk about the group to others, talk about yourself and what you are learning. If at any time you become unsure that confidentiality is being respected, bring this matter up in the group. If you do not feel trusting because you are afraid that others will talk, this doubt will surely hamper your participation.

• • • • • • • • • • • • • • • • • •

Depending on the type of group you are leading and the nature of the membership, you can formulate your own written list of suggestions for maximizing the group experience. It helps to have a list that members can keep and review periodically. Some group practitioners might argue that it is better not to provide a list because members should struggle to find their own way. We do not agree. Our experience is that much floundering occurs when members are not given some idea of how best to do the work they came to the group to do. Moreover, we have seen group members who are psychologically wounded by hostility over their questioning, storytelling, and gossiping and who then become defensive and withdrawn for the remainder of the group. We think this outcome is unnecessary and unproductive and that it is not likely to occur if members have been told how best to participate in a group.

Preparing Leaders

In addition to preparing members to get the most from a group, you need to get yourself ready to be fully present in the groups you lead. If you do not devote time to preparing psychologically, the group is likely to suffer. In approaching a new group, for example, you might ask yourself these questions:

- How ready do I feel for this? Am I available for the members?
- Do I want to do this group? How alive and enthusiastic am I?
- How effective am I in my personal life? Am I doing what I hope my members will do in their lives?
- Am I professionally confident?
- Do I believe in the process of a group, or am I doing a group merely because I was told to?

In addition to preparing yourself before meeting a group for the first time, you can use at least some of the following procedures to get ready for an upcoming session:

- Spend some time in relaxation before you go into your group session. Reflect on what you'd like to accomplish.
- Be aware of your thoughts and feelings as you approach the group session.
- Try for yourself some of the exercises and catalysts you will ask your group members to use.
- Spend some time with your co-leader. If the two of you are not attuned, your work will be disjointed. Do you respect each other? Do you trust each other?
- Review your process notes and discuss them with your co-leader.
- Devote some time to thinking about the previous session. Where did the group leave off? How can you bridge the gap between the last session and the upcoming one?

We encourage group leaders to make frequent journal entries about themselves and the reactions that are evoked in them as they are leading or co-leading groups. Rather than describing the dynamics of their members, we suggest that leaders focus on how specific members affect them personally. We recommend that group leaders address these kinds of questions in their journals:

- How did I feel about myself as I was leading or co-leading my group?
- What did I like best about the group today?
- What most stood out for me during this session?
- How am I being affected personally by each of the members?
- How involved am I in this group?
- Are any factors getting in the way of my ability to effectively lead this group?

The use of the journal technique by group leaders provides an excellent record of patterns that are shaping up in a group. The practice of writing can also be a useful catalyst for focusing leaders on areas in their own lives that need continued attention.

Concluding Comments

In this chapter we have discussed preparation as a technique for promoting group effectiveness for both therapeutic groups and psychoeducational groups. We have emphasized screening interviews, preliminary sessions, clarification of goals, suggestions to help members get the most from a group, and ways for leaders to get ready. Many problems in the working stage of a group arise because of inadequate preparation, which results in a lack of clarity about the nature of the group and about how best to participate in it. These problems can be avoided if you develop your own preparation techniques or use some that we have suggested here.

Questions and Activities

1. To what extent do you agree or disagree with our emphasis on preparing group members? Do you think that the preparation process is essential for the success of any kind of group you may lead?
2. Suppose you are working in an agency and are asked to organize a group for a particular population. How might you go about it? Discuss such matters as recruiting, screening, selecting, and preparing members. What would you say to prospective members about what you expect of them and what they should expect of you?
3. How might you set up a long-term group differently from a short-term group? Would there be any differences in how you designed an open group (one with changing membership) and a closed group (one with the same members)? How might you prepare members differently for a psychoeducational group or a therapeutic group?
4. What is your position regarding screening members? What specific factors would you look for in deciding to include or exclude someone? How might you tell someone you did not want him or her in a group? Would you provide alternatives? If so, what might these be?
5. At this point in your professional development, what kinds of groups and what kinds of populations do you regard yourself as being qualified to lead? What groups might you be most interested in forming and leading?
6. We discussed the advantages of preliminary sessions. Can you think of any disadvantages or potential problems of such sessions?

7. Suppose a member is concerned at a preliminary meeting about whether what goes on in the group will stay there. What would you say?
8. Under what circumstances, if any, would you breach the confidentiality of your group members' disclosures? How might you explain this exception in the screening interview or the first meeting?
9. Assume that an adolescent asks you whether you would tell her parents about something she said in the group. How would you respond?
10. Think of a group that you would be interested in designing. Write a brief proposal for this group with a specific target population and present the proposal to your class. Others in the class can give you feedback on your presentation as well as on the proposal itself.
11. Break into dyads, with one person assuming the role of a candidate for a group and the other conducting a screening interview. After about 10 minutes, switch roles. Or break into triads, with the third person giving feedback. Partners should discuss how it feels to be the group leader doing the interviewing as well as being the prospective participant being interviewed.
12. Write a list of group rules that you might distribute or at least discuss with a group. Present these rules to a small group of classmates to get their reactions to your policies and to consider rules included in their lists but not in yours.
13. You are meeting your group for the first time and a member asks how he can get the most from this group. How might you respond?
14. Do you think it is important for members to clarify their goals before entering a group?
15. Some group leaders use written contracts that outline their expectations of members and what members can expect of them. What advantages and disadvantages do you see in this procedure? With what kind of group(s) might you use written contracts?
16. You discover that several members are talking outside the group about matters discussed in the group. What might you do?
17. What are your views about asking members to do reading or writing? Do you think that reading and writing are appropriate and useful for both therapeutic groups and psychoeducational groups?
18. We mention the need for co-leaders to prepare themselves both individually and as a team. What are the signs and consequences of a lack of preparation?
19. We suggest writing autobiographies as a technique to get members focused for a group. Write your own brief autobiography, mentioning critical turning points in your life and the effect they have had on you.
20. In this chapter we talk about the use of structure in groups. What are your thoughts about the balance between too much structure and not enough structure? What problems do you see with either of these extremes? Which side might you be inclined toward? Discuss.

CHAPTER FOUR

Techniques for the Initial Stage

Introduction

If a leader has done a good job in the preparation phase of any kind of group, members are more likely to come to the first session with a clearer focus and a readiness to work. The initial stage is critical because the group's identity is being formed. In this chapter we discuss some of the basic characteristics of a group during this first stage, and we provide some techniques for getting the group started and for dealing with initial resistance.

Characteristics of the Initial Stage

At the first session, both the members and the leaders have some degree of anxiety. The leaders may wonder what the group will be like, whether they will be able to deal effectively with what comes up, and whether they will be able to bring a group of strangers together in such a way that the trust necessary for effective work is created.

Members are typically anxious about not fitting in, about revealing themselves, about meeting new people, and about being in a new situation. These general fears of members are mixed with anxiety about the specific issues they intend to explore and about whether they will be able to do so. They are not quite certain about what to expect in a group, which heightens their concerns about fitting in and being accepted. They are apt to worry about whether they will be liked or disliked. Members may also be resistant, especially if the group is not a voluntary one. They may be there physically but not psychologically, they may be skeptical about the value of groups or the purpose of the group, or they may wonder how the group will be of use to them.

Even if members want to be in the group, they may be unaware of how to get involved. Is it best to be invited to speak? What can they talk about? How personal can they be? How much detail are they expected to give? How can they use the group to understand and deal with their problems? Will they behave in the group just as they do in everyday life, or will they act differently?

Regardless of the type of group, trust is a basic consideration during the early stage of a group. Members may ask themselves: "Is it safe for me to be myself?" "Will what I say be listened to?" "Can I risk revealing things about myself that I generally keep hidden?" "If I'm having negative reactions about being in the group, is it appropriate to reveal these openly? And if I do, what kind of reactions will I get from the others?"

If trust is not established in a task group, it will be extremely difficult for the participants to direct their energy to accomplishing the given task. In a psychoeducational group, if trust is lacking, it is doubtful that members will be open to learning new information and exploring the personal implications of the content that is being imparted. Members of a therapeutic group will be hesitant to engage in significant self-disclosure if they do not experience the group as a safe place. Thus, for any type of group, it is a worthwhile endeavor for leaders to devote considerable effort in doing what they can to create a climate that will be conducive to members fully participating in a way that will achieve the group's purposes and the individual members' goals.

Members are also usually concerned about outcomes. They wonder whether they will be better off after taking part. Will the group make a difference, or will it be a waste of time? Will they find out something about themselves that is unacceptable to them?

Finally, during the initial stage, people are developing roles within the group, forming alliances, testing the leader and other members, deciding whether they are being included or excluded, attempting to please the leader, and attempting to meet the expectations of other members.

Physical Arrangements and Settings

An important initial responsibility of the leader is to decide where the group will be held and to arrange this setting in a way that is conducive to group work. For all kinds of groups, some important considerations are privacy, freedom from distractions, and continuity of the physical setting. Sometimes, for example, group leaders think that meeting outdoors is appealing in good weather because of the informality, but such a setting generally lacks privacy and can be a source of distractions.

Because the physical setting contributes to the climate of a group, some degree of attractiveness is necessary. If the meeting place has no windows and is poorly ventilated, if it is cold, or if it is uncomfortable, attention is bound to be drawn away from exploring personal issues. In a clinical setting or hospital ward, if the walls are bare, or the group room sterile and uninviting, the leader can encourage the members to think of some imaginative ways of brightening the atmosphere. This technique helps members get involved.

Seating arrangements are important. A group that meets in a room where members are physically separated by tables or otherwise spread out has a different quality from a group that meets in a setting that promotes eye contact and allows for some closeness. When a member cannot see all the other members, when some members are in corners of the room, when some are sitting behind others, and when other physical barriers are present, psychological distance and fragmentation can be expected. By the same token, when members are too crowded together, closeness is forced on them. Another consideration is that an atmosphere that is too comfortable and informal can foster inattentiveness. Although the considerations pertaining to physical arrangements may seem obvious, leaders can easily overlook such matters.

In the sections that follow we discuss techniques for getting groups started. In using these catalysts, you might listen for the themes mentioned in the earlier section on characteristics of the initial stage and use them as clues in deciding how to proceed.

Getting Acquainted

Introductions are one of the first items of business for any type of group. Depending on the kind of group, a variety of approaches can be tried. Also, whether the group is an open one or a closed one determines some of the techniques that are best used in helping members get acquainted. In a group where members come and go, obviously, it is crucial that new members be introduced as they enter.

Learning names. One technique is to have people introduce themselves by name and say anything about themselves they would like the group to know. Before members start, they are asked to repeat the names of all those who have introduced themselves previously. In this way members can learn one another's names in a few minutes by sheer repetition. Our preference is to avoid going around mechanically in a circle. We encourage the members to bring themselves into the group without being called upon by us. By asking members to spontaneously bring themselves into the group, we gain some information about them. This practice also keeps the process of getting acquainted moving quickly, as members are anxious to speak up before the list of names to be remembered gets too long.

Introducing oneself. Consider asking members to introduce themselves in different ways. For example, they might introduce themselves as the people they'd like to be at the time of their final session. This technique gets people to think about their goals. It gives others a sense of what each person hopes for from the group, and it gives all a chance to begin taking risks. Leaders can ask members to say more about themselves than they normally would when they first meet others. This technique provides a way for members to decide at the outset how much they are willing to be different in the group.

Here are a few examples of other catalysts that leaders can use to help members begin to get acquainted:

- Could each of you make a brief statement about how it was for you to come here today? What were you feeling? What were you thinking?
- What do you expect this group to be like for you? What do you hope it will be like? What do you fear it will be like?
- How did you find out about this group? What were you told about the group?
- What do you most hope you'll learn in this group? What are you willing to do to get what you want?
- What are some of your fears about being in this group?
- Why are you here? Now that you're here, how is it for you?
- What previous experience have you had in counseling or in groups? What did you learn about yourself from these experiences?
- Is there anyone else who wants you to be here? How is that for you?
- What is a major struggle in your life at this time?

Introducing someone else. Another technique for getting people introduced consists of asking members to pair up and get to know as much as possible about their partner so that they can later introduce the partner to the entire group. Partners should avoid bombarding each other with probing questions. They can instead be active listeners and can share as much about themselves as they choose to. This technique gives members practice in speaking about themselves to one other person. The exercise typically takes about 20 minutes. The leader can announce when it is time to switch from listener to speaker. Otherwise, quiet people may spend the entire 20 minutes in polite listening and say only a few words about themselves. Before the reverse introductions begin, members can tell their partners what, if anything, they do not want the group to know. As a variation, instead of introducing each other, members can say what it was like for them to listen to their partner. If this is done, however, it is important that members avoid putting the focus on their partner or telling specific details about the partner. Instead, what is important is that members tell how *they* were affected.

Setting a time limit. You can ask members to relate the aspects of themselves that they deem significant in not more than three minutes. Members can share something of their past, focus on their current lives, or express their future hopes. They can also share whatever they are feeling at the moment. This is a good follow-up technique to the previous one, because it gives each member an opportunity for self-presentation. You can begin this process by introducing yourself. It is best that members not react or respond during this go-around. Discussion can follow after everyone has had a turn. This technique will often provide you with ideas for later use. You can note especially how members use their allotted time. Some run over in an attempt to convey as much detail about themselves as possible, whereas others quickly run out of things to say and are embarrassed.

Using dyads and small groups. The use of dyads is appropriate for both psychoeducational and therapeutic groups. To lessen members' feelings of being intimidated by a large group, you can ask them to form dyads or triads for about 10 minutes and get acquainted with their partners. Then, they can find new partners for another 10 minutes. Depending on the size of the group and the people in it, switches can be made between 2 and 10 times. Or, after a number of changes, a dyad or triad can join with another dyad or triad and continue the exercise. This technique gives most of the participants at least a brief opportunity to make some contact with others and to say something about themselves. The use of various combinations of small groups is an excellent icebreaker and a good way to begin to generate trust and interaction within the group. Eventually, you can convene the entire group and ask members to share briefly what they experienced and talked about.

How much structure should these small groups be given? Generally, we favor bringing some focus to these subgroups, even though we allow them to deviate from discussing the questions suggested. Many psychoeducational groups are structured around a particular theme or topic, and it can be useful to ask members to form dyads or small groups to share their thoughts and personal reactions to a topic that will be explored in a given session. The advantage of encouraging discussion of particular issues or topics is that the entire group can later focus on certain themes. It also encourages members to take an active rather than a passive role. Any of the questions we suggested in the section on introducing oneself would be appropriate here.

The use of subgroups entails the risk of fostering permanent alliances. Therefore, you might check to be sure that the membership of subgroups changes frequently. If alliances do form within the group, this needs to be talked about.

The leader's role. A leader's task is to keep things moving in the initial go-arounds when people are introducing themselves. This enables everyone to have several opportunities to make statements, and there is no sustained focus on a single individual. It is a good practice to discourage members from asking questions, especially about why people feel as they do. If a question-and-answer format is established at the beginning, it can continue for the entire course of the group. To keep the focus moving from person to person, leaders often find it useful to have a number of go-arounds, asking several of the questions we suggested. Members who tend to be quiet can be encouraged to participate. Asking only one question at a time lessens the chances that members will feel overwhelmed.

Leaders can be actively involved in the introduction process in order to begin to establish trust. They can share their feelings about starting the group, say what they expect and hope for, tell something about their experience in leading groups, and, depending on the particular group, disclose something about themselves personally. They can add what they gain from leading groups and what they hope to learn or experience in this group. Remarks about what they are aware of at the moment are often the most valuable, because such disclosures model a focus on sharing present experiences for the members.

Focusing Members

Paying attention to the group process. It is important for the group facilitator to teach members how to pay attention to the group process, even in psychoeducational groups with a teaching and information-giving agenda. For example, if participants are talking abstractly about a particular theme, chances are that others may have a difficult time staying involved. Content can best be imparted and shared if there is receptivity within the group.

As therapeutic groups begin to take shape, it is important for leaders to pay attention to the subtle aspects of the emerging group process and to teach members how to recognize their own reactions. At the first session we sometimes ask members to quietly size up everyone in the room. We encourage them to silently focus on their assumptions, reactions, and perceptions regarding each individual. We always stress that we will not ask them to reveal these reactions at this time. Our purpose is to assist the members in clarifying some of the thoughts and feelings they have as they are put into a new group of people.

During the initial stage of most groups we make a concerted effort to teach members how to pay attention to their own behavior in the context of what is occurring in the session. At the first session we frequently ask "What is it like for you to be in the group? What are you most aware of? What are your expectations?" As members are making themselves known through the process of "checking in" or saying at the beginning of a group what they want out of it, we silently take note of their style of speech and their use of metaphors. As the group is just beginning to evolve, we rarely interpret the members' use of language; rather, we take note of it and look for patterns and connections if they continue to develop over time.

At the second meeting of a group, we often begin by asking each member to check in by addressing some of the following questions: "Who were you aware of as you were going home last week?" "Who were you thinking of and what were you thinking about as you were coming to the group this morning?" "What most stood out for you about your experience in the group last week?" "Did you have any reactions about our first meeting during this past week?" Our basic purpose in presenting this line of questions is to teach members the importance of paying attention to the ways in which they are affected when they are in the group and to underscore the importance of expressing persistent thoughts and feelings.

During the initial phase we frequently remind participants how important it is that they not keep their reactions to themselves. We tell them that our concern is not with what they *say* but with what they keep to themselves. For instance, if members are aware that they are frightened of speaking out because they are intimidated by the group leaders, it is imperative that they let this fear be known.

Focusing on issues outside the group. We have indicated the emphasis that we put on harnessing the group's energy in focusing on the here-and-now interactions within the room. Paying attention to how members behave in the group situation tells a good deal about their behavior outside of the group. Indeed, we find that if we are successful in getting members to deal with their here-and-now experience of being in a new group, it frequently leads them to reveal the pressing concerns in their daily life that brought them to the group in the first place.

We also employ techniques that assist members in focusing on issues outside the group. Our techniques have the general purpose of enabling members to talk more concretely about themselves and less about other people in their lives. If they do talk about others, we encourage them to say how they are affected rather than merely giving detailed stories about others. We employ open-ended questions such as these to get members focused on outside issues that they want to explore in the group:

- If your life now is as good as it gets, would you be OK with that?
- If this were your last opportunity for therapy, what would you want to work on?
- What in your life is a source of concern for you?
- What stops you from pursuing the goal you have identified?
- What are some specific thoughts or beliefs that tend to interfere with your functioning as effectively as you might like?
- If there were just a few specific behaviors that you could modify, what would they be?

Creating Trust

There is no single technique or even a set of techniques that alone creates trust. As we emphasized in Chapter 1, as the leader, you are your most important technique. The kind of person you are and your ability to establish direct contact with others are likely to be major determinants of the level of trust in your groups. Using techniques without first establishing a good relationship with group members is likely to result in suspicion and holding back on the part of the members. Such a relationship is best established by paying attention to the needs of individual members, responding to them in respectful ways, appropriately self-disclosing, being willing to state your expectations openly, encouraging members to talk directly to one another and doing so yourself, being sensitive to the fears and anxieties of the members, and providing people with opportunities to openly say whatever they are feeling or thinking.

In the initial stage a basic task of a group is dealing with mistrust. Mistrust takes several forms. Members may mistrust themselves. They may ask themselves: "Do I trust myself enough to look at what is going on in my life?" "Am I trusting enough to express my feelings?" Members may also mistrust other members. They may have negative reactions to some members that contribute to their hesitation in making themselves known. Finally, members may mistrust the leader or co-leaders. Although some participants may naively have an automatic sense of confidence and trust in group leaders, others may have initial reactions of mistrust and cynicism because they perceive leaders as authority figures: mothers, fathers, police officers.

The issue of trust is never settled once and for all and will continue to manifest itself in different forms throughout the time the group is together. We tell members that their trust may rise and fall. Furthermore, we don't think it is necessarily a bad sign if group trust diminishes. It is essential, however, that the members demonstrate a willingness to acknowledge their lack of trust. Members need to learn that the more threatening the material explored becomes, the more the issue of trust is central. Certainly the delicate nature of trust is a focal point for the early stage. We continually let members know that trust is not something that merely happens to them; rather, it is the outcome of the risky steps they are willing to take to bring this level of safety into their group. We emphasize that a good place to begin is by talking about what makes it difficult for them to feel a sense of trust in one another.

The leader's most important task in dealing with mistrust is to give members many opportunities to talk about their feelings early in the group. If work is to proceed, mistrust must first be recognized and then dealt with in the group. If it is not, a hidden agenda develops, the lack of trust is expressed in indirect ways, and the group grinds to a halt. If a basic sense of trust is not established at the outset and the group leader tries to push an agenda too soon, serious problems can be predicted: lack of enthusiasm, little energy, and awkward silences.

A hidden agenda—an issue that is not being acknowledged or openly discussed in a group—can sabotage any group. For example, in a training group in a master's program, a hidden agenda may emerge around honest self-disclosure if members think they will be evaluated on what they share of themselves in the group. Even in a committee formed to accomplish a specific task, a hidden agenda can develop if the members of that committee have different purposes from the stated objective of the group. In any kind of group, conflict that is not recognized and dealt with in a sensitive and effective manner often results in a hidden agenda. The real issue does not get talked about, which results in the group getting stalled in its progress.

Consider the following example of how a hidden agenda during an early session can temporarily inhibit the trust level in the group. Rashad had expressed considerable emotion during a session, and many members seemed involved in his work. On returning the next week, however, the members seemed more guarded than they had been the week before, and there was a mood of quietness in the group. With the prodding of the group leader, members eventually revealed what was behind their hesitation to speak up. Some were frightened at the intensity of Rashad's feelings. They were not sure what they should do about the reactions they had. Some did not want to interrupt his work, but they were very aware of being deeply touched by him. Some who were moved personally were afraid to acknowledge this for fear that they might "lose control" as Rashad had. Although some members wanted to get involved by discussing their own problems, they put the brakes on themselves for fear that they would be inappropriately interrupting what he was doing. Other members were angry because they felt that he had been "left hanging." They couldn't see what good it had done for him to get so worked up and then not get an answer to his problem. Still others eventually confessed that they were burdening themselves with "performance standards." They thought that to be accepted in the group they would have to display a great deal of emotional intensity. They were afraid that if they did not cry others might perceive them as being superficial.

All of these reactions are material for possible productive interaction if the members are indeed willing to bring them up. By fully expressing and exploring such reactions, members genuinely develop the basis of trust. On the other hand, if members stifle their reactions, the group loses its vitality. Those group issues that do not get talked about almost always develop into a hidden agenda that immobilizes the individuals and the group.

You can recognize when a climate of trust has been created because members then express their reactions without fear of censure and being judged, are actively involved in the activities in the group, make themselves known to others in personal ways, take risks both in the group and in everyday life, focus on themselves and not on others, actively work in the group on meaningful personal issues, disclose persistent feelings, and both support and challenge others in the group.

By contrast, here are some signs that trust may be lacking:

- Participants are slow to initiate work.
- Members say very little when called on for their reactions.
- Members keep negative reactions to themselves, share them only with a few, or express them in indirect ways.
- Members deflect by telling detailed stories.
- Participants intellectualize.
- Members are vague and focus on others instead of on themselves.
- There are long silences.
- Participants put more energy into "helping" others or giving others advice than in sharing their personal concerns.
- Some maintain that they do not have any problems that the group can help them with.
- Others are unwilling to deal openly with conflict or even to acknowledge the existence of conflict.

When trust is lacking, members sometimes make judgmental statements, which have the effect of inhibiting open participation. For instance, a member may say to another person: "You're acting! You never talk about yourself. You're always judging everyone else." Or another member may express a feeling of being judged by asserting: "If I don't say it just the right way, I will be criticized. There is just too much attacking in here. I'm afraid of this group."

So far we have stressed the components of building trust that cannot be replaced by exercises. We have emphasized paying attention to the relationship that the leader is developing with members and that the members are developing with one another. Once members have been encouraged to express their lack of trust, trust can be encouraged by using techniques that foster a sense of community. We present here a few techniques that facilitate the process of establishing trust and security within a group.

Identifying fears. The anxieties that participants have about themselves, other members, and the leader or co-leaders can be explored as one way to generate trust. If these fears are kept secret, they are simply magnified and continue to grow. If they are acknowledged openly, they are likely to subside or at least not inhibit participation in the group.

We try to help participants explore their fears. Oswaldo indicates that he is afraid of this group experience. The leader asks Oswaldo to close his eyes and imagine the worst thing that could happen to him in the group. (Closing the eyes helps members focus on internal states and block out external stimuli.) Oswaldo says, "I think the women are going to think me foolish." The leader asks him to elaborate. He says that he fears being verbally attacked by the women present. He imagines that he will not know how to respond, and that he will become paralyzed, will cry, and will look stupid. The leader says, "Oswaldo, would you open your eyes now and look around the room to see who you most worry might respond to you in this way." Oswaldo identifies Rita. The leader encourages him to elaborate on this fear, and, later, encourages him to seek out feedback from Rita and the others on what he has disclosed. These sorts of techniques allow members to express their fears openly instead of letting them fester inside unacknowledged. We find over and over that what causes problems in a group is not the feelings and thoughts people do express but those reactions that they do *not* express.

Dealing with fears. As a leader you have a number of ways of working with fears once they have been identified. Let's suppose that Sothea says, "I'm afraid of being myself in here, because I don't know how people will react to me." She can live out this fantasy in the group by imagining how different people will react to her. She can also see herself leaving and having the worst feelings possible. Sothea can be asked to make the rounds and say out loud, in a few words, what she guesses each person might say to her. This method allows her to face some of her fears by exaggerating them and imagining the worst possible outcomes. Another approach is simply to let her talk about her fear in the group. She may admit that she has this fear in most social situations and so avoids new situations. Another technique is to have all those in the group who share Sothea's fear form an inner circle. They can talk about the ways in which they behave similarly and about how they deal with their fears.

Another way to deal with mistrust is to ask participants to imagine what it would take for them to feel secure enough to reveal significant things about themselves. Some may say they would want to know that they were not alone in what they felt; others may say they would want some assurance they wouldn't be attacked by others; still others may add that they would need people who cared and were supportive. Members can also break into dyads to discuss what inhibits their ability to trust and what it would take for them to be more trusting. Then, when the whole group reconvenes, the leader can ask members to talk about what they said in their dyads and what they learned about creating trust. Giving participants time to explore their fears contributes to the building of trust. In talking about their distrust, they are helping to create trust.

Another trust-building exercise after people have been together for at least a couple of sessions and have had some opportunity to formulate some impressions of one another is to ask them to look at each of the others in turn and ask themselves: "How is it to be in the group with this person? Am I willing to be open with this person?" Or participants can ask themselves: "With whom in this group do I feel the closest? From whom do I feel the most distant?" After a few minutes, you can ask whether anyone is willing to report any reactions. We want to avoid putting people on the spot and do not pressure them to give their reactions. Instead, we leave it up to the members to decide if they want to give their reactions out loud. This device brings out into the open reservations that participants might have, and it can facilitate a discussion of how members are being affected by one another. If members are having doubts or reservations about others, these reactions need to be acknowledged and openly dealt with if trust is to be established.

Physical trust-building exercises have a different flavor from the techniques we have been advocating. For example, in the blind-trust walk a member is blindfolded and led by another. This exercise forces the "blind" individuals to trust their guides to keep them from stumbling. Some find it exhilarating to relinquish control and have confidence in another.

Although physical exercises can be worthwhile, we rarely use them. In the kinds of groups that we have done, we find that trust develops slowly through facilitating the group's own struggle toward trust. Our preference is to facilitate trust by encouraging participants to express their internal fears. Doing so challenges them to work with what they are honestly feeling.

Addressing Initial Resistance

One of the best ways of developing trust is to recognize the beginning signs of resistance. Resistance is a natural and healthy part of the group process. Regardless of how highly motivated clients may be to get involved in their group, awkwardness and tentativeness permeate the atmosphere until people begin to get a sense of one another. As a group is forming, we expect participants to have reservations in revealing aspects of themselves that they generally do not freely share with strangers. They have good reason to feel threatened, for the unknown does not inspire a sense of security. Resistance is not simply lack of cooperation, and not all resistance is negative. A better term for resistance might be "reluctance." Members are likely to be reluctant for a variety of reasons and a good way to create a safe climate is to invite members to talk about any reluctance they may be experiencing. After all, it is to a great extent healthy to be cautious about making oneself known until it seems safe to do so. Thus, reluctance, or any form of resistance, is not something to be avoided or bypassed.

Pretending that resistance does not exist will not make it disappear. Ignoring both obvious and subtle signs of resistance leads only to a group's becoming bogged down. Blaming the members for being stubborn and unmotivated is likely to increase their defensiveness. Blaming yourself for your ineptness as a group leader does not help. Resistance can be constructively explored only by encouraging participants to state some of the factors that are keeping them from getting involved and by acknowledging these sources of their hesitation.

Being sensitive to fears. An obvious source of resistance in the initial stage of a group is pushing participants too quickly to overcome the fears and anxieties that are normal at this stage. Members' fears can be compounded if they volunteer extremely emotional and traumatic material early in the group's history. It is critical for leaders to be sensitive to this possibility and to patiently explore the here-and-now fears and resistances that are an inevitable part of a new group. As tempting as it might be to focus on a member's disclosure, this could be frightening and overwhelming to other members. Leaders do well to assist members in pacing their disclosures.

We would not try to stifle one member's emotional revelations about a recent loss, but we might try to pace it so members are not pushed into doing work for which the group is not yet ready. If one person introduces herself to the group with an angry tirade about her partner, rather than trying to draw this out at this time, we might comment on how we hope she will let us return to this later in this session. The idea here is to facilitate the expression of all these themes but also to establish some pacing for the group as a whole.

Modeling. A good technique for overcoming resistance in the initial stage is modeling by the leader. When you are experiencing resistance from members, you can give your reactions without blaming them. If there are many silences during an early session, for instance, you might say any of the following:

- What makes it difficult to talk in here?
- It seems to me that some important things are not being said in here.
- I hope each of you says something about what you are aware of right now.

As a leader, you can talk about how the resistance affects you, and you can invite members to say what they are experiencing. Such modeling encourages members to express their feelings and is an important and direct way of dealing with any resistance that is brewing in a group.

Working with involuntary groups. Resistance can be a special problem in groups composed of involuntary clients. Here we briefly discuss resistance as a characteristic of clients who are required to attend a group, and we describe some techniques for dealing with this resistance in a therapeutic fashion. Too often leaders assume that not much will occur in involuntary groups because members are forced to attend. This attitude is easily communicated to and picked up by the members. The opportunities for significant change in such groups should not be overlooked.

In general, people who come to a group as a condition of parole, as a part of treatment in a mental health facility, on the order of a judge, spouses who come under threats of divorce, or adolescents who are sent by their parents or the school are somewhat closed. Techniques may emphasize acknowledging understandable resistance and also illuminate constructive opportunities the group may afford.

One place to start with in working with clients who do not initiate treatment is to challenge the attitude of being an involuntary member. In most instances, members do have choices. For instance, an adolescent who is sent to a group can refuse to attend and face the consequences that she may be expelled from school or face reactions from her parents. Even in these "involuntary" situations, there are choices. Choices have consequences, but they are choices nevertheless.

Before attempting to do any significant work with the problems members may have, it is crucial that leaders explore the attitudes members bring to the group and what they have been told about the group. Members probably haven't been told much about how groups function or about what they might gain from participating. Thus, they have a cynical attitude and a passive style of resisting. They may say little and expect to be questioned. We think leaders can educate these members as to how they can use the group to get clearer about what they do want and how they might go about getting it.

Members who exhibit reluctance may have some of the following thoughts and feelings:

- I'll say as little as possible.
- I'll be very careful about what I say in here so that it can't be used against me.
- They might be able to get me here, but they can't get me to talk.
- Why should I trust these leaders? They've never been in my shoes.
- I can't see why I should let anyone in here know what I'm thinking. I don't need them.
- This is just another game.
- I'm here to satisfy my partner, but I can't see how this will help me.
- This therapy stuff is stupid. Talk never changes anything.

If members who display resistive attitudes or behaviors are encouraged to verbalize these thoughts, the words they use can provide material for inventing a technique to explore the resistance further. For example, the member who says "I'm going to say as little as possible" might be asked these questions: "How are you going to do this? How will you keep things to yourself?" Another member can be asked to say more about how others are likely to use things against her. The person who thinks the leaders have never been in her shoes can be asked to talk about what she sees in the leaders that convinces her that they will not be able to share her experiences. The person who says that talk never changes anything can be asked to identify some things that matter to him that talk is not going to change.

Leaders should identify resistance in a group and then work to make it explicit. In doing so they are training the group members to express themselves, and they are helping establish a climate of trust because they are communicating to clients that they understand and respect their resistance and are willing to work with it rather than trying to argue it away. In a subtle way this technique reduces resistance because members who came determined not to talk are now talking. Leaders should be careful to present the technique in clear language, with a minimum of jargon.

A potentially useful device is simply to allow the members to express openly for a time their feelings about being forced into a group, without comment from the leader and especially without the implication that they shouldn't feel that way. This technique is a good one to use at the beginning, because it may be the first time that anyone has shown them respect, which can be the basis for building trust. Eventually the leader can begin to deal with the feelings of resentment, hostility, helplessness, and defiance by saying, "Now that you have expressed these feelings, what can you do about them?" This leads the group beyond complaining and prevents the meeting from becoming merely a gripe session. It can also be the start of rapport.

Another way to respond to resistance in clients who are required to attend a group is to make brief contacts with them individually and to spend some time getting to know them. Clients, especially those who live together and attend the group as a part of a treatment program, frequently have had no orientation. They are merely told to attend. A brief contact or several contacts outside the group can be the beginning of rapport.

A direct technique for use in a session is to encourage questions about how the group will function, what the leader's role will be, and related matters. Some members may assume that whatever they say will be recorded and perhaps used against them. You can help establish trust in this situation by being honest about your role in the group and about how much of what goes on in the session you will report. For example, if you are required to keep notes on clients and put a summary of their progress in a file, you can assure members that you will discuss with them what is going into their folders. Or you can role-play what you are going to say to supervisors about clients.

A basic approach for working with involuntary groups is to inform members that, although they must attend the sessions, you are open to suggestions from them, and they will have a significant impact on how the time is used. You can then point out some possibilities. Members who come to a group reluctant to do more than put in their time may find value in attending if alternatives for using that time are explored. Also, members should have an immediate opportunity to evaluate the group. Resistance can often be lessened when members are encouraged to assume some responsibility for how the group functions.

Another freedom sometimes available to involuntary clients is not to participate in a session. If this is a fact, this can be turned into a technique. They are obliged to be there physically, but they can form an outer circle where participation is not required. If they change their minds, they can join the inner circle, which is a working group. There may be some limitations to the use of this technique. For example, the institution may not allow it, or the working members in the inner circle may object to being observed by the silent members.

Starting a Session

We have talked at length about preparing members and getting a group started, but we also want to give some attention to ways of starting a particular session. When a group is in its initial stage of development, we typically begin each session with at least one go-around. The practice of teaching members to briefly check in permits everyone to have some sense of what others are thinking and wanting. If we quickly focus on the first person who speaks and do not wait for others to check in, we often miss potential themes and ways of linking members with common issues. We may repeat our encouragement for everyone to check in before moving on to develop any one theme or to work with any one member. Here is one way of inviting members who are hesitant to speak up to check in: "It helps to hear your voice early on. The longer you wait to speak, the more difficult it is going to be to participate. Even if you think that you have nothing to say, it helps to hear your voice."

Leaders may expect that group members will arrive ready to begin work, but it's generally helpful to spend a few minutes getting focused. It is sometimes useful to facilitate connections between sessions, especially with work left unfinished at a previous session. In a typical go-around, members declare what they want from this session and whether they wish to discuss anything left over from the last meeting. Leaders may ask people who disclosed important material at the previous session whether they had reactions during the week to their disclosures or have further thoughts about what they did. This technique provides an opportunity for linking sessions and for following up on clients. Leaders must be ready to intervene if members get too detailed in their process of checking in and clarifying how they would like to use time for this session. If leaders do not intervene, it is very possible that most of the session will be consumed by the checking-in exercise. Leaders need to be alert during the initial go-around to avoid interventions that invite people to become emotionally involved. Surely this process of briefly checking in must be sensitively handled, and members often need the leader's guidance in getting to the point.

The following remarks indicate other ways of getting a group focused:

- What do you most want from today's session?
- I'd like to have a go-around in which each person completes the sentence, "Right now I am aware of _______."
- Close your eyes, realize that the next two hours are set aside for you, and ask yourself what you want and what you are willing to do to get it.
- If your best friend were to introduce you in this group, what would that person be likely to say about you?
- Do any of you have thoughts about last week's session or any unfinished business from then that you want to bring up now?
- What would you most want us to know about you?
- How would you like for this session to be different from the previous one?

- What were you aware of as you were getting ready to come to the group this afternoon?
- What fears or doubts do you have about this group?
- When you think about this group and how it has been for you, are there any aspects that you would like to change?
- Last week some of you said that you felt forced to be here. How are you feeling about that now?

Ending a Session

During the first few sessions, it is a good idea to spend some time asking the members to say something about how they view their participation. We discuss issues and techniques for ending sessions in more detail in Chapter 7, but at this point we describe bringing closure to the first few sessions. Questions such as the following are useful catalysts for assisting the members to say a few words about what has been most meaningful to them:

- What are a few things that you think you're taking away with you from this session?
- Are you seeing any of your concerns reflected in others as they talk?
- What are you finding to be most helpful to you in here? And what is least helpful?
- Are there any ways in which the group can help you feel more secure in here?
- Was there anything that you didn't say earlier in this session that you'd like to briefly say before we quit?
- Are there any ways in which you'd like to be different in the next session than you were today?

It is useful to shape the practice of getting members to reflect on what is occurring within the group. Even eliciting a few words from each person about the highlights of the session provides the pulling together that is so necessary as the group is taking shape. Avoid ending abruptly with little or no closure.

Even during the initial sessions, members may get involved in work and feel as though they don't have enough time to finish what they started. If a client's work has been interrupted either because the group ran out of time or because the client was distracted and lost momentum, the leader can help the member briefly state what he or she would have liked to accomplish. This sets the stage for returning to this work at a following meeting.

Members need to learn that they will rarely "finish" with a problem they bring to the group, for there are always new facets of most issues to pursue. For example, the leader might say, "You know, Sariah, tonight I thought you were just getting started talking about your divorce, and we are running out of time. Is that something you would like to come back to next week?" Maybe Sariah says, "I did feel unfinished, but I think that the feelings are gone now." Here the leader may encourage Sariah by asking this: "Even though the divorce topic may seem no longer present, you have said that you feel unfinished. Are you willing to return to it at the next session?"

Continuity for dealing with problems that members have introduced in a prior session can be sustained for the next session even if the client believes the opportunity has been lost. The leader can ask the client to start in again at the point where the interruption occurred, perhaps prompting with specific phrases. Without forcing the issue, leaders frequently find that the feelings return readily enough if the client will only begin speaking.

At the first few meetings, it is an important task for members to learn how to use the time they have allotted. Perhaps some of them will come to see that they wait too long before identifying a concern they'd like to pursue. Toward the end of a session the leader can teach a few brief ways of putting their personal agenda in clear terms and asking for time. Even during the initial stage, it is well for leaders to begin teaching members how to evaluate what they are giving and getting from their group. The last few minutes of a session can be devoted to some form of verbal or written assessment of that particular session. We now turn to ways in which members can best participate in this process of evaluation.

Member Self-Evaluation

Early in the course of the group, the members need to learn how to assess their participation. The leader might ask any of these questions to help group members assess their level of involvement: "How do you see yourself in this group at this time, and how do you feel about the way you are?" "If you continue being the same kind of member that you've been, how will you feel at the final session?" "In what ways, if any, do you see yourself as being different in this group than you are in your outside world?" "What are some of the things that you like best about the way you've acted in this group?" "In what ways, if any, do you see yourself as having avoided working in this group so far, and is that something you would like to change?"

These questions can be catalysts for focusing members on the direction in which they are moving. This technique invites members to change some of the ways in which they have either involved themselves in the group or remained uninvolved. If participants say that they are dissatisfied with the way they have begun in the group, the leader can help them formulate specific strategies for changing.

What about those whose participation has been minimal? Understandably, most group leaders would like to have all the members of the group participate fully—and they sometimes force the issue. For example, some call on members and ask them what they think about the topic being discussed. Others ask each person in the group to answer a question. If leaders use these methods often, members may simply wait to be called on before they respond. If nothing seems to be happening, a more helpful technique is to address this issue directly in the group. A technique that has worked best for us with members who are not involved is to challenge them to decide what they are willing to do.

A good technique for minimizing the possibility that group members will continue in nonproductive patterns is to have them evaluate their participation and progress in a group continually, perhaps by using a written form. It is a good practice to have members begin the process of self-evaluation during the first few group sessions. Then structure the group so that the participants can assess their functioning several more times. The following self-assessment form can be used for this evaluation. (An evaluation form designed for the end of a group is described in Chapter 7.)

Self-Assessment Form for Group Members

Rate yourself on the following statements using a scale from 1 to 5, with 1 being "almost never true of me" and 5 being "almost always true of me" as a group participant:

_____ 1. I am striving to be an active member in my group.
_____ 2. I am willing to become personally involved in this group and to share current issues in my life.
_____ 3. I see myself as willing to experiment with new behaviors in this group.
_____ 4. I make an effort to express my reactions pertaining to what is going on in my group.
_____ 5. I am able to talk about what may get in the way of my feeling safe in the group.
_____ 6. I am trying to let others know how they are affecting me at the time.
_____ 7 I strive to be clear about my goals and what I want from the group.
_____ 8. I listen attentively to others, and I respond to them directly.
_____ 9. I share my perceptions of others by giving them feedback on how I see them and how I am affected by them.
_____ 10. I am able to state my fears, reservations, and concerns about participation in the group.
_____ 11. I am willing to get involved in various exercises in the group.
_____ 12. I generally want to attend the group sessions.
_____ 13. I am able to provide support to others without coming to their rescue.
_____ 14. I take an active role in creating trust in the group.
_____ 15. I am open to considering feedback in a nondefensive way.
_____ 16. I seek to carry lessons learned in the group into my outside life.
_____ 17. I pay attention to my reactions to the group leaders and express what they are.
_____ 18. I avoid labeling myself and others in the group.

_____ 19. I avoid questioning others and giving them advice in the group.
_____ 20. I take responsibility for what I am getting from the group and what I am missing.

• • • • • • • • • • • • • • • • • •

When we use a self-assessment device such as this, we discuss with the group the reactions of members to specific items on the form, paying particular attention to patterns and trends in the group.

Leader Self-Evaluation

In addition to asking members to assess their progress in the group during the initial stage, leaders and co-leaders can evaluate their own effectiveness in the group at this time. The following form can be used at different times during the life of a group for self-assessment and also as a springboard for fruitful discussion between co-leaders.

• • • • • • • • • • • • • • • • • •

Self-Assessment Form for Leaders

Rate yourself on the following statements using a scale from 1 to 5, with 1 being "almost never true of me" and 5 being "almost always true of me" as a group leader:

_____ 1. I am generally enthusiastic about meeting my group.
_____ 2. I am willing to express my reactions to what is going on in the group.
_____ 3. I am able to help members clarify their goals and take steps to reach them.
_____ 4. I am able to understand members and to communicate this understanding to them.
_____ 5. I can challenge members in a direct way without increasing their defensiveness.
_____ 6. I am able to model desired behaviors in the group.
_____ 7. I am willing to take risks in pursuing hunches I have in working with members.
_____ 8. My timing of techniques is usually appropriate in that it does not interrupt the client's work.
_____ 9. I am sensitive to picking up clients' leads and following them rather than pushing members.
_____ 10. I am able to challenge my initial assumptions and perceptions regarding members.
_____ 11. My behavior in the group indicates that I have a basic respect for the members.
_____ 12. I am able to link the work of one member with that of another by picking up common themes.

_____ 13. I give thought to what I want to accomplish before I enter a session.
_____ 14. I allow adequate time for a summary and integration at the end of each session.
_____ 15. I am able to intervene effectively with members who engage in counterproductive behavior without attacking them.
_____ 16. I provide support and positive reinforcement to members at appropriate times.
_____ 17. I usually work effectively with my co-leader, and when I don't, I am willing to admit it and talk about it at the appropriate time.
_____ 18. I make use of appropriate self-disclosure.
_____ 19. I use techniques with sensitivity to the client's cultural background.
_____ 20. I give thought to the techniques that I use in a group and have some rationale for using them.

• • • • • • • • • • • • • • • • • •

Concluding Comments

During the initial stage of a group, the following are key tasks for leaders: to create an environment that helps build trust; to deal with members' fears, anxieties, and expectations; to be aware of their own persistent feelings and reactions; to encourage members to express persistent feelings and reactions regarding the group; and to help members go further in expressing personal reactions than they typically do. The early phase of a group is critical, because at this time the norms that will govern the group process are being shaped and the foundation of trust is being laid that will allow for productive work as the group moves forward. This early stage is particularly vulnerable to leader-created resistance, perhaps more so than at any other time. It is crucial that leaders convey the message that they are there to work *with* the members rather than "on" or "against" them. Members watch leaders very carefully to determine if this is a safe place. If the members' fears and reservations are not dealt with effectively as the group begins, the members are certain to encounter obstacles to developing genuine cohesion that will unite them. They will inevitably be stuck if they do not explore the fears that can keep them from fully participating.

Questions and Activities

1. How would you describe the characteristics of the initial stage of groups with which you are familiar? What techniques are you likely to use at the beginning of a group? What are your reasons for introducing these techniques?
2. Describe circumstances under which you think icebreaker techniques are in order. Describe techniques you might use to help members get

acquainted, and give your reasons for introducing them. What potential disadvantages are there to using them?

3. Examine the room you are in right now. How might you best use this room for a group meeting? What are its liabilities, and how could you maximize its potential as a group setting?
4. How does the body posture of members influence you in a group? How would you avoid misinterpreting body language?
5. We have said that structure is more appropriate at the initial stage of a group than later on. Do you agree?
6. After reading this chapter, which techniques did you find most interesting for use in the initial stage? Why?
7. What are some possible advantages or disadvantages in using exercises to create trust?
8. In the early stage of a group, do you favor using some structured exercises, or do you lean more toward letting the group find its own way? Does your answer to this question depend on the specific type of group you might lead? Discuss.
9. You are asked to lead an involuntary group. Describe how you would deal with the issues you imagine would surface in the group, and discuss what techniques might be appropriate or inappropriate. How would you explain to the members the potential value of the group?
10. Enumerate several characteristics of resistance and the possible dynamics behind them, and create techniques that you think might be appropriate for working with them.
11. How can you differentiate between a member's reluctance to trust that arises from cultural conditioning and resistance that stems from avoidance?
12. At the first meeting of a group, a member declares that you do not have the experience or ability to be leading. How might you deal with this challenge?
13. What techniques can you think of to get members focused at the beginning of each session?
14. How would you go about evaluating your own effectiveness as a leader? Describe some specific procedures.
15. What are some of the ways in which your modeling can lessen resistance among the members? What kind of modeling would you like to present when dealing with resistant behaviors?

Guide to Using *Groups in Action: Evolution and Challenges* DVD and Workbook

The first program, *Evolution of a Group,* illustrates real-life examples that often occur during the initial stage of a group. After viewing this initial segment of the program consider these questions:

1. *Characteristics of the initial stage.* Think about how characteristics of the initial stage of a group are depicted in the first program. For instance,

what are the members anxious about, and how safe do most of them f from the very beginning? Do some members feel as though they are o. the outside?

2. *Techniques for getting acquainted.* What techniques are used to help members get acquainted? What use is made of dyads? How do members learn each other's names?
3. *Techniques for focusing members.* Some members believe their cultural differences might be a factor in their feeling a part of the group. How do the Coreys deal with the issue of cultural diversity, which emerges early in the life of this group? What specific norms are the Coreys actively attempting to shape early in the group?
4. *Techniques for creating trust.* Issues of trust are never settled once and for all. Think about the fears of members that may lead to low levels of trust in this group, and answer these questions:
   - How would you describe the level of trust during the initial stage?
   - What are some techniques the Coreys use to establish and maintain trust early in the life of this group?
   - What are some specific fears that the members raise? How are these fears dealt with by the other members and the co-leaders?
   - What did you learn about some ways to create trust in a group through viewing the early phase of this group?
5. *Techniques for dealing with initial reluctance.* Resistance (or reluctance) is not simply lack of cooperation, and not all resistance is negative. What specific manifestations of reluctance do members show during the initial stage of this group? What are some of the reasons members had for displaying resistive behavior, even though they are motivated and are participating in the group voluntarily? The co-leaders of this group must deal with conflict during an early session. What can you learn from this interchange concerning how to deal with conflict between members? Members are also asked to share what might get in their way of participating effectively in this group. How can this question help members identify ways they are likely to resist?
6. *Opening and closing group sessions.* Notice the use of the check-in and the check-out procedures in the DVD. What techniques would you use to open a session in a group you are leading? What did you learn about leader interventions in getting members to check in and state how they would like to use time for a session? What specific techniques for ending a session did you read about and also observe in the DVD? What are some lessons you are learning about the importance of bringing a group session to closure?
7. *Using the workbook with the DVD.* If you are using the DVD and workbook, refer to Segment 2 (Initial Stage) of the workbook and complete all the exercises. Reading this section and addressing the questions will help you conceptualize group process by integrating the text with the DVD and the workbook.

E

ues for ansition Stage

Introduction

In this chapter we discuss some of the basic characteristics of a group during its transition stage. We focus on therapeutic ways of working effectively with defensiveness and resistance and provide some techniques for dealing with a range of problematic behaviors. We also discuss how to deal with members with whom we are having difficulty. In some places, we link certain techniques that we describe to a specific theory underlying the practice of group counseling. As much as possible, the therapeutic rationale for the technique being described is explained.

Characteristics of the Transition Stage

Before a group can launch into deeper work, typically it goes through a transition phase that can at times be very challenging. In early phases of a group, there may be a sort of "honeymoon" where members address significant issues in their "outside" lives but avoid being very direct with one another in the group. Later, the group will hopefully come to have a greater ability to work both on outside issues and on members' experiences of one another. This transition period is often characterized by conflict. This may be thought of as a kind of testing ground in the development of the level of trust. Members may voice criticisms of one another and, often, of the leaders. It is important to take these criticisms seriously while also understanding their place in the larger process. We think of this transition stage as a positive move toward greater intimacy, but members may be dismayed that the honeymoon is over. It is very important for leaders to have an understanding of this very normal era of conflict, and we caution against using techniques that ignore or try to override significant issues. Techniques can be introduced, however, to illuminate and to expand on what is taking place.

At this evolutionary period, members and leaders have the task of learning to recognize and deal with anxiety, resistance, and conflict. The members may be working through any (or several) of these issues:

- Deciding whether they are willing to invest themselves fully in a group experience
- Becoming explicitly aware of feelings of which they were previously only dimly aware
- Testing both the leader and other members to determine the safety level of the group
- Observing the leader's behavior to determine the congruence between what the leader says and does
- Feeling ambivalent about what they want from the group
- Becoming more attuned to conflict that might be brewing within the group
- Learning the importance of saying what they feel and think

ge, it is the members' task to monitor their feelings and arn to express them. It helps if members come to respect et, at the same time, are able to challenge their tendencies . Members are expected to learn how to confront others in tructive fashion and how to remain open and nondefensive in r back from others when they do so. If conflicts emerge, it is incumbent on members to recognize them and develop the skills to work through them. Unrecognized conflicts will almost always lead to hidden agendas that can result in a group becoming stuck.

A central challenge for leaders at the transition stage is to develop interventions that help the group become a cohesive unit. Techniques need to be used with sensitivity and appropriate timing. One of the leader's tasks is to encourage members as they go through some difficult times. At the same time, leaders need to challenge members to face and resolve conflicts that evolve from the interactions in the room. At this juncture, it is critical that leaders' actions be consistent with their words. If leaders expect group participants to be honest, direct, and constructively confrontive, it behooves them to model these behaviors. Perhaps the most critical behavior a leader needs to model at this time is respect and protection for a member who may be scapegoated because he or she presents an unattractive persona. For example, a member who is acting angry may be very hurt. Or a member who appears arrogant may really be shy or frightened. Additionally, a member who is scapegoated may be serving the group's need to keep intimacy at bay. Some members are liable to become the scapegoats for a group's need to direct conflict onto one person so as to create resistance. Although it may be true that a member has been intellectualizing, or monopolizing, or judgmental, the group may be overstating the trait they insist this individual displays. Consequently, while applauding this movement toward honest exchange, the leader must be prepared to protect the scapegoated member by describing to the group the process the leader believes to be at work. Techniques that bring the focus back to the members having the reactions, with less focus on the potential scapegoat, may be best here.

Dealing with Defensive Behaviors

It is sometimes tempting to refer to individuals as "difficult members," but we avoid addressing people in our groups in that way. From our vantage point, we do everything possible to avoid labeling people and to give them a chance to be different. We aim to be patient even though their behaviors may strain our patience. We attempt to see various problematic behaviors as signs that people are struggling, and in this spirit we strive to understand what purpose their behavior is serving. In this section we provide examples of defensive or avoidance behaviors common to the transition stage of a group and explain how to work through some of these difficult situations.

Having an external focus. Members in the transition stage of a group frequently focus on other people and on matters external to themselves. They may blame others either inside or outside the group for their inability to trust. For example, Darlene announces that watching Charlie sitting back and looking bored makes it difficult for her to be invested in the group. Instead of looking at herself and her reactions, she focuses much of her attention on what he is doing, what he is not doing, and how she thinks he is "making" her feel. In this way she avoids dealing with her lack of involvement in the group.

One technique the leader might use here is to ask Darlene to speak directly to Charlie and tell him how she is affected by his presence in the group. If Darlene says "Charlie is so aggressive," the leader might ask, "What does his aggressiveness, as you see it, do to you?" If Darlene is responding to Charlie as she does to someone close to her, perhaps she might reply: "Charlie, I'm scared of you, and I find myself reluctant to open up around you. You remind me of my ex-boyfriend." With this, we might say, "Before you focus more extensively on your feelings toward your ex-boyfriend, would you be willing to talk more to Charlie about how he is affecting you and how it might be for you to open up more personal feelings relating to your ex-boyfriend." Our rationale here is to make sure that we facilitate a process in which Darlene can feel safe. Lingering feelings of Charlie scaring her might inhibit her ability to become emotionally vulnerable. This technique of directing the focus toward clients who are making statements about others tends to encourage members to look at themselves and their part in the group. This creates the kind of dialogue we hope to have in the working stage. At this stage of the group's development, we want to address the reactions members have toward others in the group.

In working with Darlene, we are influenced by the psychoanalytic approach to group therapy. The concepts of both resistance and transference are especially relevant in this situation. By placing her attention on Charlie's behavior, Darlene does not have to recognize aspects of her own behavior. She also gives us a clue that transference may be operating in that she may be projecting feelings she has toward her ex-boyfriend onto Charlie. A psychoanalytic way of working with transference is to actually foster these feelings so that Darlene can eventually recognize how unfinished business with her ex-boyfriend might be playing out in her present relationships and in her interactions in the group. In the therapeutic setting the leader and other members would not criticize or judge Darlene for having or expressing the feelings she has about Charlie. When Darlene's feelings are accepted by group members, she can begin to understand how old feelings may still be operating in the present. The psychoanalytic approach gives us a useful perspective on resistance, projection, and transference (see Corey, 2004, chap. 6).

Using impersonal and global language. John characteristically speaks in general terms and thus keeps himself shut off from other members. During one of the early sessions, the leader asks members to tell how they feel about being in the group. John says, "Nobody in here really wants to open up. Everyone is sitting back and waiting for the other person to begin. People are not saying what they think. They don't want to step on anyone's toes. Nothing is happening in here, because everyone is putting up walls, and nobody wants to come out from behind these walls." Because John uses universal terms such as *nobody, they,* and *everyone,* others in the group have no idea whom he is talking about. Also, it's not clear whether he is including himself in this category because he doesn't say that he has walls or that *he* is unwilling to open up. Here are some possible interventions the leader might use to help John become more personal and use more precise language:

- John, I'd like you to say everything you've just said, but put "I" in front of each of your sentences and see how that sounds to you.
- How about going around the circle and completing this sentence in a different way as you look at each person: "One way you could help me in this group would be _______."
- Tell us some of the ways in which the situation in this group seems like situations you find yourself in outside the group. How are you the same both in the group and in daily life?
- Could you replace each of the remarks you have made about other people's walls with a comment about some wall of your own?

The rationale behind having John participate in any of these interventions is for him to get past his projections. We are interested in having him put the focus on himself rather than on others. One theory explaining the dynamics of projection in a group is Gestalt therapy (see Corey, 2004, chap. 11). During the transition stage, when issues such as the struggle for control and power become central, projection continues to be a primary style of interacting. From a Gestalt therapy perspective, conflicts that occur at this stage are difficult to resolve unless the members who are projecting their needs onto others eventually recognize what they are doing.

Other techniques for helping members narrow down their generalized statements are also useful. Here are a few generalizations we have heard in our groups, followed by interventions we are likely to make in an attempt to help the member become more concrete and focused:

Member: "People are cautious about opening up."
Leader: "What are you cautious about in here? If you were to be less cautious right now, what might you say or do?"

Member: "Why do we always have to talk about problems? Why can't people ever talk about the positive things in their life instead of always focusing on the negative?"
Leader: "What particular problems are you reacting to? How would it be different for you if the members did not talk about problems?"

Member: "Why is it that unless you cry or get angry you are not believed?"

Leader: "What has it been like for you to be in this room when members cry or get angry?"

Member: "My problems are not as significant as other people's!"
Leader: "What problems of yours do you consider insignificant? Whose problems in here are more significant than yours?"

The art of skillful leadership involves confronting members in such a way that they will be more inclined to recognize defensive patterns such as focusing on others or consistently keeping themselves hidden by using impersonal and global language. Confrontation is not limited to a few theoretical orientations; it is part of most of the major contemporary theories of group counseling. When confronting members, describe specific behaviors and do not criticize or label members. When used in this way, confrontation can be a valuable tool for exploring resistance.

Asking questions of others. A particular form of avoidance behavior that often manifests itself during the transition stage is asking questions of others. This defense, if unchecked, drains away the energy from a group. Members using this defense demand that others make themselves known while they are hidden behind their questions. For example, Jim perceives himself as an active and involved member merely because he asks a lot of questions. Even though the group is relatively young, he has already managed to ask personal questions of most of the members. He has asked others to give reasons for the feelings they have, and he has asked them whether they have tried this or that approach to solving a problem. His questions have usually interrupted group interaction.

Keeping in mind that Jim's style of questioning is a way of avoiding focusing on himself, the leader can ask Jim to talk about what prompts him to ask questions or to address what he hopes to get from members by questioning them. In this way, Jim can begin to disclose something of himself.

Questions are not always manifestations of resistance. The types of questions that we would like members (and leaders) to refrain from asking are leading questions, questions that pry, or questions that are closed-ended and tend to cut off a member's exploration. Questions that come from a place of compassion and concern seldom pose a problem. Questions asked merely to satisfy curiosity are rarely helpful.

Returning to Jim, suppose Jim comes under attack from others in the group who take their clue from the leader's intervention. Now they start to berate Jim for his endless questioning. The leader might, at this point, propose a technique in which Jim is encouraged to state his own concerns, which may be hidden behind his questions. Alternatively, Jim's critics might be asked to elaborate on their own previous experience with feeling overly interrogated. So far, the leader's suggestions are aimed at giving some direction to the conflict in ways that are honest yet not needlessly attacking. Perhaps matters take another turn here. Jim, and a few others, now confront the leader on having a double standard for who should or should not ask questions. When the leader is the "lightning rod" for transition stage conflict, it is paramount not to hide defensively behind yet more techniques, which can serve to deflect reasonable criticism. At the same time, the leader may do well to ride out the storm with the realization that this, too, is a typical sort of transition stage event.

Dealing with Members Who Display Difficult Behaviors

Members display certain difficult behaviors most conspicuously in the transition stage, and the leader's early responses to them set the tone for the group. Members are observing the leader's behavior and are often silently deciding how much they can trust this person. In this section we discuss participants who are sometimes troublesome and give suggestions for dealing with them.

General principles. It is a mistake for leaders to label some struggling members as difficult members. This is judgmental and illustrates a common error of dealing with content rather than process. Additionally, what we consider to be difficult behavior in a member may really be a leader's countertransference. Leaders are sometimes unsure whether their reactions to an individual are valid or are rooted in their own idiosyncracies and unresolved conflicts. In general, we assume that our personal reactions to group members genuinely tell us something about the members and about ourselves. For example, if we find ourselves chronically annoyed with a certain behavioral pattern that Roberto displays, it may well be that he is repeating an old and familiar pattern that has been characteristic of his interactions with people since his early childhood. But it may also represent struggles in our own lives.

Although it is likely that Roberto is exhibiting transference in the group, his behavior may well be triggering reactions in other members and the leader. In fact, his behavior may be inviting people to shut him out or to dismiss him. These patterns are typically replayed in the interactions within the group, and we can learn a great deal about his dynamics by tuning in to our reactions to him. The feedback from other group members can add to our understanding of Roberto provided we are not lulled into being convinced that we are right.

The perceptions we have of our clients are in many ways our best tools and the source of our techniques. For this reason we allow ourselves, with some caution, to be guided by them. However, countertransference reactions are often rooted in our own unfinished business, and we had better come to terms with our sources of vulnerability so that we do not get locked into a nontherapeutic alliance with a client we perceive as being problematic. If we do not become aware of our unresolved conflicts, then our reactions can interfere with the group process. Our willingness to explore our countertransference provides us with significant clues to the dynamics of both our clients and ourselves. The psychoanalytic orientation to group therapy offers a template for understanding how transference and countertransference patterns may be operating in a group (see Corey, 2004, chap. 6).

The greatest responsibility of a leader is to facilitate insight and change. To do so, the leader cannot rush in too quickly with attempts to change members or "cure" them of their difficult behaviors. Initially, the leader should gather data, ascertain whether the members see themselves as causing problems for themselves or others, and discover what they might be attempting to communicate through their behavior. Both other members and the leader must be patient and nonjudgmental if resistance is to give way to more constructive behaviors. Those who exhibit problematic behaviors in the group can usually be dealt with in a direct and caring manner and can be given more of a chance to change in the group than they might be given in daily life. The basic purpose of a therapeutic group is to provide people with opportunities to see themselves in a new light and get a more accurate picture of how others perceive them. In the group context they can learn that they do not have to persist in a behavioral pattern that is leading them in a direction they do not wish to pursue. With the security afforded in a group, they can open themselves to taking risks and can dare to be different.

Leader modeling is extremely important here, for members do learn through this process. A common danger is to sum up members too quickly by attaching labels to them such as "monopolizer," "group nurse," or "seductive one." Such labeling may entrench these behaviors and motivate members to retreat defensively into the identity given them. If members who exhibit resistive behaviors are subjected to undue pressure or to uncaring attacks, the group can actually have a toxic effect rather than a therapeutic one.

A general guideline for leaders is to avoid saying, "You are difficult" and to say instead, "I am having difficulty with you." Leaders can then point out specifically how and why they are being affected the way they are. For example, rather than saying, "You're a storyteller, and by telling stories you're being a bore," the leader might say this: "When you go on in such great detail about another person, I have a hard time paying attention to you. I'd much rather hear how you're affected by this person." Or the leader might express to the member: "I'd really like to be able to stay present with you and understand you, but it's not easy for me to get a sense of you when you describe things in so much detail."

When members know a specific behavior that others have difficulty with, they can learn to observe this behavior in themselves. Then they are in a position to decide whether the behavior is a problem to them and also whether they are willing to change it. A member who typically loses others by going into extraneous details may decide not to change this behavior, but the member must be willing to accept the reality that this choice has consequences.

If leaders initiate feedback about a troublesome behavior, they can do so in a manner that is sensitive, honest, nonjudgmental, and caring. Others in the group are likely to be observing their manner of confrontation, and thus it is well for them to be aware of what they are modeling for the members. For example, if most members see Doug as unapproachable and let him know this, they can be encouraged to provide Doug with their feedback and reactions but avoid ganging up on him. The leaders need to be careful to moderate the amount of feedback so that Doug does not get more than he can possibly assimilate at any one given time. If it appears that he is getting more feedback than he can handle from others, the leader may intervene by saying "Perhaps Doug has enough to think about right now. Maybe we can focus more on what is going on with each of us." To offer an opening for further work, a leader might add, "Before we do that, Doug, how was it for you to get all this feedback? Do you have any response to any of the feedback that you have received so far?"

Although members exhibiting challenging behaviors may experience any sort of feedback as criticism, it is nevertheless best for you, as the leader, to support the right of others to voice their reactions. However, you might also communicate strong supportive interest in and caring for the recipients of the feedback through your acceptance, patience, and willingness to stay with them. Your task as a leader is to help members see and understand the difference between critical reactions and helpful reactions. You might let members know that the feedback from others, ever so hard to hear, may be coming from a caring place. You can ask members whether there is anything they would like to try doing differently or whether there is further work they would like to pursue.

When a member hears all feedback as a criticism and an attack, you might ask in a supportive way, "What did you hear said to you that felt like an attack? Would you address the members who you felt attacked you and give them some idea how they could give you feedback that would be more helpful to you?" If a member is really locked into the notion that she is being attacked, it may well be that at this moment there is no way to talk to her without her feeling attacked, no matter how caringly it seems to be done. Rather than pursuing this issue at this time, it may be more helpful if she would be willing to reflect on the feedback that has been given to her. Another approach might be to ask the member who feels attacked to address different members and tell them how she needs to protect herself from what they are saying. She could be asked to complete an unfinished sentence such as "I need to protect myself from you because _______." People who have difficulty with confrontations may at some point become so overwhelmed that they truly shut down. Stop further confrontation because such confrontation is no longer therapeutic. A leader could suggest that members write down their afterthoughts and feelings.

We don't give recipes for working with members who demonstrate difficult behaviors in a group. Your own reactions and inventiveness have to be the guide. It is important for both the leader and the members to talk about themselves when they are having difficulty with a member. Rather than focusing on judgments or interpretations of behavior that you perceive as being difficult, talk about how you are affected in a personal way by these behaviors. In this regard, your ability to be honest, sensitive, caring, and timely is of the utmost importance. Often, it may be inappropriate to introduce any explicit technique at all beyond encouraging feedback and individual expression and offering interpretation of or comments on the group process.

In the transition stage, the group has not yet achieved the cohesion necessary to work on problems at a deeper level. Thus, it may be inappropriate to promote much in-depth work with a difficult member who has received confrontive feedback. Even if this person is now ready to express some emotion or to work on some difficult and threatening material, the others in the group may not be ready for this work and may be excessively frightened by what they see as the consequences of giving feedback to one another. As we mentioned, the early interchanges with members who exhibit problematic or difficult behaviors should be seen primarily as a source of valuable information for you to use later on. For example, you may want to ask certain members whether the responses they elicit from the group match the responses they get in everyday life or that they got in childhood.

The group setting provides an excellent format for people to see their own resistances in action. If members can avoid labeling themselves and putting themselves down in critical ways, they are more likely to feel the freedom to try out a different form of behavior. Techniques for working with members who display problematic behaviors fall into two categories: those that focus on the member and those that focus on the responses of others to this member. Either focus can flow into the other, and you should be alert to this possibility. Techniques that focus on resistive behaviors include having members receive feedback to clarify the impact they have on others; having them exaggerate their behavior, perhaps to see it clearly, to tire of it, or to gain insight into its sources; having them try out a different behavior; and having them talk about how it feels. Techniques that focus on the responding members include asking them to comment to the member who behaves defensively in this way: "When I feel your defensiveness, I am reminded of _______."

During this kind of work, be alert to the danger that group members will label difficult clients or that these clients will label themselves, particularly when they feel defensive, and then live up to these labels for the duration of the group. If leaders steadfastly refuse to reduce people to some sort of stereotype, the members themselves are less likely to continue self-labeling. One of the purposes of a group is to provide a context in which participants can challenge self-defeating labels and begin to create positive identities. Techniques that invite members to experiment with new forms of behavior are especially useful. In this way, members can not only think about ways in which they have embraced a limiting vision of themselves but also learn from the experience of trying something different.

One way of stimulating members to consider changing their behavior is to ask them whether they're getting from the group what they had hoped for when they signed up. If there is a discrepancy between the goals they have stated and how the leaders or the group members are seeing them, they can be invited to examine the discrepancy. In this way leaders can check whether the members themselves want to change. Are they interested in feedback? Do they think that they may be restricting themselves by accepting self-imposed labels or the labels others have given them? Do they want to take the risks involved in creating a different identity? If they decide that their current behavior is not working for them and they want to change it, the group is an excellent place for them to learn constructive behavioral changes.

Before suggesting specific techniques for dealing with group members who display resistive patterns, we want to underscore some key points. Whom you experience as difficult depends on *you* as well as on your clients. You can trust your reactions while also acknowledging that these assessments reflect on yourself and on your own dynamics. You can communicate your own responses to members who behave defensively and can model this kind of feedback for other group members. Try to communicate a basic respect for the clients whose behaviors pose difficulties, even though the feedback given to them may be critical. Most important, be alert to how this kind of feedback may entrench clients in their problematic behaviors. Communicate to these group members your openness to them as they are now and encourage them to consider experimenting with ways of being different as a means of obtaining the goals they stated when they came to the group.

The person who is silent. Leaders need to model respect for members who are silent if they hope to create a climate that invites rather than forces members to participate. At the same time, it is important for leaders to communicate their interest in hearing from members who are hesitant to verbally participate and to be aware of the impact that these members may have on others in the group. Other members may eventually comment on those who are not participating, and these quiet members may appreciate this interest. If leaders initiate the topic of silence, they can ask members to evaluate whether the group is productive for them. If it is not, they can encourage hesitant members to discuss what is inhibiting them. They can also inform these members of the impact they have on others, particularly when others seem to be inhibited for fear of being judged by those who do not participate. Finally, leaders can express an interest in whether the silence exhibited by these members is indicative of their style outside the group, and they can remind members of their opportunity to try out a different way of being if they really want to change.

Both group leaders and the other participants can make the mistake of pushing members who are silent to open up without discovering why the person is being silent, and they can make the mistake of focusing on the member and using any means of drawing out this individual. As a result, the member who tends to say little often becomes increasingly quiet and withdrawn. In many cases, silence is not a defense but a learned behavior that is congruent with the client's cultural background. For instance, Quan says very little in her group. Despite repeated attempts of other members and the leader to get her to say more, she remains a polite listener. Eventually the group discovers that in Quan's culture it is considered rude to talk about oneself; doing so would be seen as being self-centered. Thus, when she asks questions of others, she is doing what works for her in her family and larger culture. After a while, she lets the group know that she does not judge others for talking in very personal ways about their families but that for her to do so is most difficult. She has been taught that it is shameful to expose the family's personal matters in public. Quan does tell the group that she does not like being seen as "the quiet one" in so many social circles. She states that she appreciates people who are outgoing, and she would like to become a bit more outspoken—but it is difficult for her due to her cultural upbringing.

A technique for exploring the reactions of active participants to one who is silent is to encourage them to tell one another or the member who is silent (depending on how threatening the leader judges this to be) how they feel about having expressed themselves openly around someone who has not reciprocated. Exercises of this type can be introduced in a way that minimizes embarrassment to those who are typically silent. In the case of the verbally disclosing members, the emphasis is best placed on asking them to reveal how they are affected by a member's silence. Active participants can complete a sentence such as the following: "For me it is important that you speak up because _______." We cannot give a blueprint for what is appropriate here. You may want to be more confrontive with someone whose silence is manifestly hostile, disruptive, and manipulative. You will likely want to be more supportive with someone who is shy or inhibited.

A technique for working with several members who display silent behavior is to ask them to form an inner circle and then to say as much as they are willing to about their being silent. They can be asked to talk about what it has been like for them to be in the group so far. The chances are that they have been very observant and that they can share openly what they have been thinking and feeling. The leader needs to make sure that these people are interested in doing the exercise.

A variation of the preceding technique focuses on the members who are active. They can form an inner circle and talk about their feelings about not knowing what the members who are not participating are thinking. This exercise gives those in the inner circle an opportunity to discuss how it is for them to disclose in the presence of those who do not. It also gives those who are verbally inactive (in the outer circle) feedback about the impact of their silence on others.

As a further illustration of possible techniques for dealing with the member who is habitually silent, we now describe Donna's behavior and apply some of the principles we have just been discussing. When the leader asks her how she has experienced the group so far, she shrugs her shoulders and says this: "It's hard for me to talk in a group. I prefer being a listener. I don't like feeling forced to talk and to say what I think. I learn a lot just by listening to what others in here are saying." One approach is to ask Donna whether she'd like to be different from the way she is. Would she like to be more verbal in the group? Is her listening style satisfactory to her? Is she getting what she wants by being silent in the group? Such questions are typical of the reality therapy approach to group counseling. Members are encouraged to look at their present behavior to see if it is getting them what they want. After making a self-evaluation of their behavior, members are in a position to make changes if they discover that what they are doing is not working for them. Reality therapy in groups offers a variety of specific procedures that can lead to change (see Corey, 2004, chap. 15).

Using another approach, the leader can say something like this: "Donna, I want you to know how powerful an impact your silence has on me. For example, I find myself imagining how you might judge the way I'm leading this group." Or the leader can ask Donna to talk about what it is like for her to be in the group or what she is thinking about members who have spoken up. How does it feel for her to be a listener? How is her behavior characteristic of the way she is outside the group? Is she aware of what keeps her from saying what she is thinking and feeling in the group? By answering these questions, Donna is letting people know something about her.

Donna may eventually say that she talks little in the group because she doesn't know what is expected of her, that she has never been in a group before, and that she'd like to say more but finds herself being inhibited and doesn't want to call attention to herself. She may say that the others seem to know what they want from the group but that she still doesn't know what to work on. One technique to use here is to ask Donna to look at each person in the group and complete the sentence: "When I look at you, I think you expect me to _______." She may complete the sentence with one of these phrases: "talk as much as you do," "come up with some problem to work on in this group," "become involved in this group or decide to leave," "tell you that I'm not judging you and that I accept what you're saying," "show some feelings," or "tell you something about myself." Donna's statements provide rich material for the leader to tap into. After she has made the rounds and dealt with her projections, she can be asked what this experience was like and what she learned from the exercise. Then members may want to spontaneously offer her feedback about their expectations of her. It is important not to short-circuit the process of Donna's struggle. If she were to say, "I wonder what people think of me, and I wonder if I'm living up to what others expect of me," we would generally not facilitate by encouraging members to share their reactions too quickly. We prefer her to work with her own projections and her own internal dynamics before she seeks reassurance from others.

Another technique for working with expectations is to focus on Donna's expectations of others. She can go around the group and complete the sentence "Looking at you now, I expect you to _______." These two exercises can be combined by asking her first to go around the group saying what each person expects of her and then to go around making statements about what she expects of each person. (This is a Gestalt experiment described in Corey, 2004, chap. 11.)

If Donna lets us know that her silence is something that troubles her and that she would like to change it, we can ask her to talk more about how it has been for her to be in this group up to now, having said little. We can invite her to pursue any of these questions: "What are some things you're thinking and telling yourself when you want to participate but don't?" "How do you imagine this group might be different for you if you were to say more?" "You say you've been silently observing and learning. Would you tell us what you've been learning? Perhaps you could address specific people in here, letting each of them know what you're learning from them." Any of these questions could facilitate Donna's work in understanding the ways in which she inhibits herself. She can begin to see the functions her silence serves.

A final suggestion for working with Donna is to ask her to close her eyes and imagine that the way she has begun the group—namely, assuming the role of listener—is the way she will continue until the end of the group. She can be directed to imagine that this is the last session. What is she thinking now? What has she gotten from the group? How does she feel about her level of participation? What might she be saying to herself? This technique is designed to get her to think about the pattern of behavior she is developing in the group and to project this pattern into the future. (This is a form of the future projection technique used in psychodrama, which is described in Corey, 2004, chap. 8.)

This technique gives Donna a chance to examine how she may be allowing expectations that she imagines others have of her to interfere with her participation in the group, and it gives her a chance to declare what she is willing to do differently if she doesn't like what she sees when she closes her eyes.

The person who monopolizes. The member who is silent is likely to be challenged by the group, but the person who monopolizes group time is often less likely to be effectively confronted. Some leaders prefer to let group members struggle in their own way with a member who monopolizes. If you prefer having a group in which many take an active role, however, you may choose to intervene. Here again a technique may not be called for; simply sharing your observations and reactions may suffice. Techniques that draw out the reactions of others are appropriate here because those who monopolize are already getting plenty of time. You should guide this feedback to guard against inhibiting the talkative individuals. You can say that those who speak a lot are valued for what they are contributing and that you hope they will continue to be active, however, you will want to challenge other members to speak up more. A powerful technique to use with clients who monopolize is to videotape or audiotape their work. By providing this direct feedback, members can evaluate how they present themselves. In addition, highly structured techniques such as using a stopwatch or an egg timer can be helpful.

Another technique that may be useful with individuals who tend to monopolize and with other members who exhibit difficult behaviors is to recommend that they persist in their behavior. Thus, saying "I'd be interested in seeing what would happen if you talked more often" may have the effect of reducing their talkativeness. You can then comment on this response and explore it. But this approach would need to be gauged against the potential outcomes for a particular member and the trust level of the group. The rationale here is that by exaggerating a style of behavior the members may gain increased awareness of what they are thinking and feeling at the times when they talk a lot. If they gain this self-awareness, this could open up possibilities for them to explore what they are attempting to get from others by putting the attention on themselves continually.

A client who is problematic is often able to assimilate feedback that is given caringly, but humorously. For example, sometimes a member may spontaneously give a good-natured imitation of a monopolizing individual. However, a word of caution is in order here. If sufficient trust has not been established, there is likely to be a boomerang effect. The person who is getting the feedback may feel put down and exhibit another equally problematic behavior or may increase his or her monopolizing behavior.

The person who habitually focuses on others. Members who do not give of themselves and who avoid talking in personal terms often cause difficulty in a group. This category includes self-appointed group leaders, those who seek to bandage the pain of others without allowing them to explore it, those who constantly offer advice, those who question others endlessly, those who assert that they no longer have the problems others are struggling with, and those who offer advice gleaned from their experience. All these members tend to give the impression that they have no struggles of their own, thus providing a less-than-supportive environment for those who are trying to be open about their problems.

Like the members who are silent, these clients are likely to be challenged by others in the group. It is a good idea for the leader to encourage other members who are feeling inhibited to express and work with their reactions. This feedback in itself is often all that is needed to cause members to focus on themselves. In addition, leaders can teach group members that, paradoxically, we sometimes give more to others when we let them profit from the time we take for ourselves than when we direct our attention to trying to help them directly.

These techniques are not intended to take away from members a sense of altruism or a desire to help others but to show them that the group is seeing only one side of them: their need to give advice, to give comfort, or to take care of others. These members can be reminded of their stated goals to treat the group as a place where they can get something for themselves, where they can learn to receive from others, and where they can decide whether their giving style is working for them or whether they might not profit from adding other dimensions to themselves.

One technique for encouraging change is to ask the member to go around and give each person one piece of advice and then to say, "And from you I want _______." This technique allows the client to do what comes easily, which is to give advice. It also asks the client to do something difficult, which is to ask for something from someone else. Of course, this technique works only when the member wants to at least consider changing the type of behavior being described.

Dealing with Conflict

A transition stage characterized by conflict and the expression of a variety of negative reactions is often observed as a group develops. Many conflicts result from the failure to deal directly with members who exhibit difficult behaviors. If a group is to make progress, conflicts must be recognized and dealt with openly.

As resistances are manifested, it is essential to understand the purpose and function that these behaviors serve. During the transition stage, members often challenge one another and are challenged by the leader. As a part of the group's striving toward its own independence, leaders are also frequently challenged, as you will see later in this chapter.

Intermember conflicts. The following are comments that members might make during the transition stage:

- I think Florian is intimidating.
- I don't like all this hostility.
- Why do we focus so much on the negative?
- Some people are monopolizing the group time.
- There's a lot of intellectualizing going on.
- I don't belong here because my problems are not as severe as those of everyone else.
- I'm bored.
- We're not talking about real issues.
- Some people sound as if they have it all together.
- I have a hard time opening up around Lawrence because he reminds me of my boyfriend.
- Drew is slouching and looks bored.

These remarks are, for the most part, indirect, focused away from the speaker, and negative. Your response to virtually all these statements might be designed to change indirect confrontation to direct confrontation. Encourage members to replace "some people," "he," and "she" with a personal focus on themselves. Suggest that Dima tell Lawrence about herself and how she responds to him rather than telling him how he is or who he is.

The group must experience and work through this stage rather than retreating to insincere politeness, but how conflicts at this stage are handled is extremely important. A group often finds a scapegoat and directs excessive and unconstructive negative feedback to that individual. One technique here is for leaders to direct attention away from the scapegoat by giving feedback to the group as a whole, describing the nature and stage of the group process as they see it, and commenting on the importance of struggling with the emerging conflict in an honest way. It is also useful for leaders to make personal rather than judgmental statements. Here are some other techniques for dealing with conflict:

- If you're bored, what is not happening for you?
- Please tell us what you were thinking and feeling before you said you felt bored.
- Please sit directly in front of Lawrence. (Dima does so.) Tell him how you are affected by him. Now would you be willing to tell Lawrence about

experiences you have had with people in your life that he is reminding you of?

- Would you pretend for a moment that you're Drew? Slouch the way he does, and talk about your fantasy of what he is feeling and thinking, as if you were in his place.
- Would you like to say, Florian, how it feels to be told you are intimidating?
- You claim you don't belong in the group, Toni, because your problems are less severe than those of the others. Please tell each member of the group how you differ from him or her. Afterward, I'll invite them to express their feelings about what you've said.
- Dima, you said your father was very critical. Would you role-play him and continue with your criticisms of Lawrence in the way he would phrase it?

In the last example the leader's response is fairly interpretive and is inappropriate unless the surrounding context is right. Furthermore, this intervention tends to take the focus away from the conflict in the room. It could be appropriate at this stage, however, because it could lead members to explore their individual dynamics when expressing their reactions to others. Also, it is clearly fitting to ask a client to elaborate on associations if the client has already indicated that this connection exists ("Lawrence reminds me of my boyfriend").

In general, leaders need to check out the reactions of the client receiving the criticism but work primarily with the person giving it, partly to teach members that they are in a group chiefly to explore and express themselves rather than to change others. What a leader models at this point can stimulate the group's progress. A leader can demonstrate the difference between "telling Lawrence who you think he is" and "telling Lawrence how you are affected by him." We prefer that members talk about how they are affected by Lawrence rather than telling him how he is.

In addition, the leader can give Lawrence an opportunity to say how he feels about what has been said to him. If he seems resistant to this feedback, the leader can emphasize that she hopes he will consider what was said but that he need not accept it. She needs to be alert to the group's haranguing him or trying to force their feedback on him and could comment that the group members may have found a scapegoat instead of keeping the focus on themselves. If, however, Lawrence gives his permission for further work and is interested in exploring the validity of the feedback, the leader could encourage him to talk about how it is to be the sort of person others have suggested he is. For example, if he has been told that others experience him as judgmental and he agrees that others often see him this way or that, indeed, he is this way, the leader can ask him to exaggerate this characteristic by talking to the group in a judgmental manner. This gives him an opportunity to see more clearly that he does indeed do what others have attributed to him.

Ann, who said she didn't belong in the group because her problems weren't as severe as everyone else's, did focus on herself, but her remarks often turn out to be a disguised way of talking about others: "I don't belong here, but you folks do; I feel for all of you because you have gone through so much." Here you might first encourage her to go ahead and talk about the others—that is what is going on anyway—and then bring the attention back, more honestly, to her. For example, she may be terribly afraid of having problems like those of others in the group. Once this feeling becomes evident, you could explore this fear and related fears concerning what might happen if she allowed herself to look at conflicts in her life that she habitually glosses over.

Exploring Common Fears and Resistance

We often pick up on a sentence or a phrase and develop a technique that can help members pursue more fully a fear that could easily stop them from interacting in the group. The examples in this section explore some common fears and resistances and are linked to interventions from a variety of theoretical approaches.

"I'm afraid you won't like me." Group members are likely to feel that they will not be liked if they are candid with their thoughts and feelings. Laura prevents herself from doing productive work because she allows herself to be stopped by her fear that some people in the group might not approve of or like her. Our task is to help Laura see how she is stopping herself and to provide her with a gentle impetus to get beyond her resistance. During Laura's fourth meeting, some of the members tell her that although she has participated they do not think she has shared much of herself. Laura replies that she's afraid that if she says more she won't be liked. Another member, Noemi, observes that at times Laura seems to be looking on disapprovingly when other members talk about themselves, and as a result she feels that Laura may be judging the rest of the group. Laura says that she does indeed find herself thinking critically about other people.

Here the leader can ask Laura to voice some of her reactions to each of the members of the group and encourage her to include critical comments. In every instance Laura's remarks may be critical of the person to whom they are directed, but she may also display much insight and genuine caring. Laura can learn that she can be honest without being critical and that her honesty is appreciated. This outcome often occurs when people such as Laura voice the critical thoughts they are so frightened of. Noemi's feedback to Laura is helpful, but the leader may be struck by the fact that Noemi also seems to convey an attitude of disapproval. This is a good opportunity to pursue work with both group members at once.

There is another way to work with Laura's fear that she will not be liked. You could ask her: "Who in this room do you think won't like you? What is going on in here that makes you think you won't be liked?" The rationale for this approach is that she may sense that someone doesn't like her. She could be having a transference reaction to a particular person, and it could be facilitative to ask her, "Who do you imagine will not like you?" In working with Laura it would probably be best to focus first on who wouldn't like her and what this person might not like about her. However, the approach we would likely take would be to ask Laura to answer these questions for herself and to explore her own projections. We are not likely to ask a member whom Laura identified, "Would you tell Laura what you think about her?" Furthermore, the point is not to get members to reassure Laura that they like her. Although this may feel good to her in the moment, it is not likely to be long lasting. If Laura has low self-esteem, quick reassurances will not be helpful to her in the long run. Laura needs to find ways to appreciate herself rather than looking for approval from others.

"There's someone here who bothers me." Bernie announces, "There is someone in this group who bothers me." One approach a leader might take is to say something like this: "Bernie, I'm sure what you just said has had an effect on people in this room, and I hope you won't stop there. You have made a start, so say more. Speak to this person directly and share your reactions. What is it about this person that you're having a reaction to? How does this person affect you? With all these reactions you have, you will get in your own way if you don't say more to this person directly." The leader recognizes that what Bernie is not saying will certainly inhibit both his own participation and the participation of others in the group. The leader's techniques are designed to challenge him to take the risk involved in being specific. If he does this, members can deal with him directly, and there is an opportunity to resolve potential conflicts.

"I'm afraid to look at what I'm really like." As a symbolic way of exploring Enjolie's fear of inner conflict, we might begin by saying to her: "I'd like for you to stand by that closet door over there and pretend that some hidden dimensions of yourself are inside. Maybe you could open the door just a crack, peek inside, and report to the group as you do so about what you suspect may be inside." Another intervention is to ask Enjolie to try this experiment: "Maybe you could stand inside the closet. As you peer out at the rest of us, talk about some of what you fear may be in there that you are reluctant to let come out."

There's no telling in advance where this exercise might go. People can be insightful when in a playful mood, and Enjolie may quickly identify in a half-joking manner some of the fears she has about what might be locked up inside her. Or she or others in the group may have had a childhood experience with closets—being put in one as a punishment for having expressed feelings unacceptable to their parents, for example. In either case, by encouraging Enjolie to physically move in the room to undertake this suggested activity, we make her a tangible focus of group work and feedback, a real part of the group.

Other techniques could be used here. We might ask Enjolie to list all the fears she can spontaneously come up with. She could make the list by completing these sentences: "One thing I'm afraid of is ______. And this reminds me of another thing I'm afraid of, which is _______." In this form of free association we are encouraging Enjolie to identify the specific objects of her fears. Free association is a psychoanalytic technique that can be applied to group work even if the group leader has another theoretical orientation (see Corey, 2004, chap. 6). Through participating in this technique, Enjolie is assisted in engaging less in internal rehearsal and instead encouraged to spontaneously say what first comes to her mind.

"I can't see why we have to share every feeling." James makes this remark after there has been much intensity in the group. The leader can begin by finding out whether anyone else in the group has the same doubts. Those who do can sit in the center of the room and talk to one another about how they are being affected by this kind of emotion. This technique gives these people an opportunity to express some of the resistance they are experiencing, which might otherwise inhibit the group's progress, and, indirectly, it provides them with an opportunity to do the very thing they are concerned about—express some of what they are feeling. The leader can ask them afterward how it was for them to have expressed these concerns and can thus encourage them to go even further. Another way to pursue this exercise is to ask these members to talk about what they have experienced or have been taught about expressing feelings. Another technique is to set up a dialogue between members who are reticent and those who have shown some emotional intensity. After a few minutes, these people can exchange sides and try to put themselves in each other's place.

When a member like James voices a concern about expressing feelings, it is important to pay attention to several possible dynamics. James's own way of recognizing his feelings may work well for him and yet be less dramatic than the way others in the group recognize their feelings. It may be that he is expressing widespread group resistance. If so, this resistance needs to be explored. Or he may be afraid of his own feelings. In this case you might use one of the following techniques:

- When in your life might you have learned that it is better to keep feelings to yourself?
- What feelings do you find to be particularly troublesome?
- Whose voice do you hear when you express your feelings? What do you tell yourself at these times?
- If your parents were here, what would they say about the expression of emotion?
- You have seen several people here be fairly emotional. Would you be willing to tell each of them why you are hesitant to do so?
- Go to each person and speculate on what he or she would think of you if you expressed more emotion.
- Would you talk about the worst things you could imagine happening if this group were to continue expressing so much feeling?
- Suppose you decided today to keep your feelings very much to yourself. How do you picture your life 10 years from now if you stick to this decision?

Any of these exercises is likely to bring to the surface the early decisions James may have reached about the dangers of letting feelings be known. You may or may not want to explore relevant childhood lessons at this point, but when a member is fearful of the affect expressed in a group, usually you can be sure that these lessons are relevant.

Many people were taught as children to inhibit their emotions, and others witnessed devastating consequences of the expression of feeling. They may have accepted parental messages that they should not express their feelings. As children, if they dared to release any emotions, they may have met with stern reactions from their parents. In addition to what they learned from their family, they may be hearing cultural injunctions against feeling. Consequently, they may have decided to stifle all of their emotions lest they meet with disapproval from others. As a leader, if you are inclined to pursue an exploration of parental messages and injunctions, you will find theoretical support of these concepts from transactional analysis (see Corey, 2004, chap. 12). You could use techniques borrowed from Gestalt therapy in exploring childhood lessons that are influencing members today, which is illustrated in the questions in the above list (see Corey, 2004, chap. 11).

"We seem stuck in our group." Sometimes a statement made by one member seems to capture the sentiment of many. Leaders, in addition to looking at their own responsibility, need to explore the dynamics in the group itself that are slowing it down. If techniques are used at all at a point like this, the objective should be to address the reasons for the impasse and not to get things moving artificially. Our aim would be to encourage members to verbalize what they are thinking and feeling and how they are experiencing the group. A leader could create an experiment such as the following: "Maybe each of you could say a bit about whether we *do* seem stuck." Creative use of the metaphors that members voice may be helpful. For instance, utilizing the phrasing of Joanna, who says, "We seem to be stuck in the mud," the leader might propose: "How would it be if each of us commented on where we're stuck? What's the mud here? What's bogging us down?" (For more on designing Gestalt experiments based on key phrases given by members, see Corey, 2004, chap. 11.)

With or without the help of an explicit technique, it is crucial to address what is going on. A lot is happening in the group that is not being expressed. The leader knows this, but it is more productive to wait for the members to voice this. On some level the members are choosing to remain stuck. Employing any technique to reduce the anxiety in the room takes the responsibility away from the members to go beyond the point of being stuck. A better technique is simply to challenge the members to say out loud some of the things they've been saying to themselves. This approach will likely bring into the open key issues that have been hidden and should provide an opportunity for a discussion and resolution of some of these issues. Although many members may not have voiced their concerns up to this point, the leader may now hear a variety of statements from the members.

Sharon: "I'm still not willing to say too much in here, because whenever I do, people seem critical of me. So I've decided to sit back and watch."

The leader can begin by exploring with Sharon how she sees the group. She can be asked to talk about what she has been watching as well as to describe her personal reactions. She can be asked to be specific by saying whom she perceives as critical of her. This approach might provide an opportunity for the leader to discuss with the group the difference between attacking and respectful confrontation. Perhaps Sharon is defensive about even constructive confrontation. Or perhaps the leader or some of the members are being overly aggressive. This technique allows the leader to discover whether the block is within Sharon or whether this is a block for most members. If confrontation is generally being handled poorly by the group, the leader needs to both model and teach a more effective way of confronting.

Janice: "I'm afraid to let myself get involved because I don't want to cry. If I begin to cry, I just might open up so much hurt that I could be depressed for days. So I'm keeping myself reserved."

Here the leader might say something like this: "Janice, could you talk about this fear of depression? Can you talk about the hurt you are reluctant to feel?" In this case, the leader is giving Janice an opportunity to either develop this material or to explain her reluctance to do so. The leader's use of Janice's words has provided a good metaphor and an empathetic connection.

Grant: "For me this group is scary. I'm afraid to open up for fear that if I do I just might go crazy."

The leader can invite Grant to explore what he imagines it would be like for him if he were to go crazy in the group. He might be afraid of becoming angry, of hurting someone, of being perceived as different, or of losing control. These more specific fears can then be worked with. Or Grant can explore his original fear in depth by disclosing to the group what he imagines it would be like for him to actually go crazy. What would he be feeling? What would others think of him? How would he deal with what he had opened up in the group when he left the session?

All of these questions are aimed at getting increased clarity of what it looks like to Grant to "go crazy." We want to find out what Grant's words mean to him and not just assume that we know. We often ask members to clarify what key phrases mean to them experientially. For instance, we know what "being crazy" looks like to us, but we really do not know what it looks like to Grant.

Dorothy: "I don't know what I want from this group. I have a hard time really deciding what to talk about when I come here. Things seem to be going pretty well in my life, and right now I'm not aware of any pressing problems I need to bring up."

She may be stuck because she no longer wants to continue with the group. She may not feel a need to explore problems, or she may not yet be able to identify specific areas of her life that she'd like to change. While it is possible that Dorothy might do well to withdraw from the group, we are more inclined to view her ambivalence as characteristic of the transition stage. Our tendency would be to ask her what brought her to the group initially and also to explore what dissatisfaction she may be currently experiencing in the here-and-now of this group's progress. All of these issues can be pursued in the group.

> Don: "Frankly, I feel we're not getting anywhere as a group because we never stick with a person long enough to solve that person's problem. What good does it do to just talk? If we're not providing solutions for problems we bring up, what good is the group?"

To deal with Don's expectation that a group is a place to solve problems, the leader could begin by asking other group members how they are reacting to what Don has said. This is a good opportunity for the group to reflect on its style or norm, which might be one of sticking with one person at a time, or more one of moving quickly from one person to another. We would also want to pay attention to Don's comments about not sticking long enough with a person's problem. Might that be a disguised message to the members or leader that he was not attended to satisfactorily?

Other members may suggest that Don is expecting simple solutions to complex problems and assert that a group's purpose is not to solve problems immediately but to give members a chance to identify personal issues and to explore various facets of these problems. Too narrow a focus on problem solving can encourage members to give advice, which has the effect of discouraging them from exploring feelings. Also, this can set off an intellectual discussion when the problem is most likely emotional.

The transition stage is an appropriate time to reexamine the purpose of a group. We can expect that members will wonder if the purpose is to solve problems, express feelings, gain insight, make behavioral changes, or simply to talk about their struggles. Will doing any of these sorts of things be useful to them in the long run?

> Molly: "So what should I do about my problem? I just don't know whether I should file for divorce or settle for the way things are in my marriage. I don't seem able to make this decision for myself, and I'm looking to the group to help me."

Molly may be feeling stuck because she doesn't see herself any closer to a decision than when she entered the group. Here is a good opportunity to work with her expectations of members and the leader. She may be hoping for outside help because she is unwilling to commit herself to a decision and accept its consequences or because she does not trust herself enough to make decisions. One way of getting her through her impasse is to have her look at the degree to which she is willing to take personal responsibility for her life. She may be using the group to justify whatever action she does take, or she may be asking the group to make the decision for her so that she will not be accountable. These issues must be explored before Molly can hope to resolve her dilemma.

In Molly's situation we are likely to be influenced by the existential orientation to group therapy. The members of an existential group are confronted over and over with the fact that they cannot escape from freedom and that they are responsible for their existence. Accepting this personal freedom and this responsibility generates anxiety, as does the risk associated with making choices (see Corey, 2004, chap. 9).

These examples illustrate that indeed a lot is going on within the group. Members are stuck largely because of their unwillingness to disclose to the group some of the things they are experiencing and telling themselves. Whenever a member speaks for the entire group, we would inevitably challenge this person by asking: "How are you stuck? How does this apply to *you?*" Our interventions are geared to getting the member who makes a global declaration about the group's being stuck to take responsibility for his or her own feelings by personalizing the statement. The basic technique here consists of encouraging people to bring out into the open their thoughts and feelings about how they are experiencing the group. This technique provides plenty of material to work with, and the group can begin to move forward.

"I don't feel safe here." Jill declares to the group that she sees others as able to openly share what they feel and talk about themselves in ways that are not easy for her. She adds that she'd like to be able to let others know what she's like, but somehow she just doesn't feel safe doing so. She agrees to work on her fears.

The leader can use a number of techniques to help Jill explore ways in which the group could become a safer place for her. One direct approach is to simply say: "Jill, I wonder whether you can tell us what it's been like in here for you? How has it been for you that you've had to hold yourself back?" These questions give Jill an opportunity to disclose what it has been like for her to be a member of the group without putting her on the spot to talk about other personal issues.

If Jill is willing to say what she has been experiencing as a member of the group, this will probably provide many leads for further work. She may acknowledge her fear of being judged by some of the members. When asked to select one of the members, she picks Peter. The leader can then say: "Jill, would you be willing to look at Peter and tell him all the things that you imagine he'd be saying to himself or to others if you were to let him know about you? It would help if you could say everything that you can think of without rehearsing. Just list all the judgments you can imagine Peter making of you." This Gestalt-oriented technique can provide the basis for a dialogue between Peter and Jill. The rationale is to give her an opportunity to say what she is silently ruminating about and to allow her to check out her assumptions. Jill may be thinking that Peter is highly critical of her, that he doesn't like her, and that he could not possibly be interested in her (see Corey, 2004, chap. 11). His actual thoughts, however, may be that he'd like to hear more from her and that he misses her participation in the group. Unless she checks out her assumptions, Jill will continue to operate as though they are true.

After the leader has worked with Jill, he might ask others in the group whether they feel the way she does. If one or more members do feel unsafe in the group, they, along with Jill, can be encouraged to tell one another all the ways in which they perceive the group as being unsafe. They can also talk about what they could do to make the group a safer place for them. Other members can then provide their feedback and reactions to this exchange.

An alternative strategy (in the style of cognitive behavior therapy) is for the leader to ask Jill to zero in on what appears to be an underlying faulty belief—that everyone is judging her and that she must gain everyone's approval—and to evaluate the validity of this belief. Irony can be used to highlight faulty beliefs. The leader can suggest that she give the group a lecture on the supreme importance of being alert to the judgments of others and on ways to gain universal approval. The leader can encourage her to say more about how it would be for her if she were not to win this approval. After her lecture, the leader can ask her to explore questions such as these:

- Who told you that it is absolutely essential that everyone approve of you? Does this assumption prevent you from being the person you want to be?
- What price are you paying to gain the universal approval you seek?
- Is what others think of you more valid and important than what you think of yourself?
- How much sense does it make to hold beliefs about others that you do not check out?

Questions such as these are based on the rational emotive behavior therapy approach to group counseling (see Corey, 2004, chap. 14). From the perspective of both cognitive therapy and rational emotive behavior therapy, clients can recognize that their beliefs and self-talk result in emotional disturbances and problematic behavior. Rational emotive behavior therapy offers a variety of cognitive, emotive, and behavioral techniques that encourage members to think about their thinking and make changes in their beliefs that are no longer functional.

Another approach consists of applying techniques from behavioral group therapy (see Corey, 2004, chap. 13). The leader may ask Jill to monitor her behavior during the week and to make notes of the times and situations in which she feels judged. She can also record what she does in such situations, what she feels, and what she tells herself. By making such notes, Jill may become aware of how her inner dialogue is creating her feeling of being judged. She can bring her notes to the group and report on the patterns of her behavior that became apparent to her. She can think about how she might behave differently in these situations and then set up role-playing situations in the session to practice specific alternative behaviors.

For example, Jill reports that she experienced much anxiety when she took her car back to a shop that had charged her $150 for poorly done maintenance. Although she was barely able to make it back to the mechanic, she quickly became apologetic and did not insist that he fix the car without further charges. Consequently, it cost her an additional $50, which she felt was unjustified. All the way home she told herself how quickly she had backed down and how her desire to gain the mechanic's approval had kept her from being as direct as she would have liked to be. In the group session, Jill can practice assertive behavior with the mechanic through role playing. Others can give her clear feedback on specific aspects of her behavior that contribute to her ineffective style in getting what she wants when she thinks she is right. The members can coach her in saying certain phrases, using a different posture, or changing the tone of her voice. Along with this assertiveness training in the group, she can also be asked to evaluate her underlying beliefs and thoughts to determine how they keep her from being the direct person she says she would like to be. This approach to working with Jill includes a number of behavioral methods: self-monitoring, behavioral role playing, feedback, coaching, and assertiveness training (see Corey, 2004, chap. 13).

This example and the preceding one illustrate that the issue of trust is not settled during the initial stage of the group. It may surface again and again and often arises following periods of intense emotion. The usual signals are silence, lifelessness, or superficiality. Leaders need to remain alert to clues that trust is, once again, an ongoing issue within the group and not a permanent state. Jill first had to deal with her lack of trust—both in herself to express what she was thinking and feeling and in others in the group—before she could openly discuss personal matters. By working on trust, she freed herself to report "failures" without being frozen by the fear that others would think badly of her.

"I can't identify with anyone here." Salvador, a retired executive, came to the group because of pressure from his wife, who complained of his being unfeeling. He rarely makes contributions in the group except to say what he thinks is wrong and how others ought to pull themselves together and be done with their problems. He usually looks critical and impatient. Finally, Patricia confronts him on this. He replies: "I can't really identify with anyone in here. Maybe it's the age difference between me and most of you, or maybe it's just that you people have different sorts of concerns than mine."

Techniques adapted from psychodrama can bring to life Salvador's own concerns. Rather than have Salvador talk about his inability to identify with others in the room, the leader can facilitate his direct encountering with others in the group. This action-oriented approach of psychodrama uses a number of specific techniques designed to intensify feelings, clarify confusions and implicit beliefs, increase insight and self-awareness, and practice new behaviors. Here are a few techniques within the psychodramatic spirit that might help Salvador experience his own feelings:

- Tell everyone in this group, Salvador, how you're different from him or her.

- Walk outside the group to intensify your sense of distance. Then talk to us about how you feel being outside.
- Pick the person you feel the most like, and tell that person how the two of you are alike.
- Now pick the member you identify with least, and tell that person how you are not alike.
- Imagine that you're driving home alone after this group meeting. Talk out loud as you reflect on how different you are from everyone in this group. (In psychodrama, this technique is known as *soliloquy*.)
- Assume that in some ways you are really very much like everyone in here. Find one way in which you could identify, even in a small way, with each person. Talk out loud as you get this picture in focus.

These techniques encourage Salvador to check out his assumptions. His lack of identification with others may be a defense. He may reveal the loneliness that results from being unable to express himself and thus identify with anyone, or he may get some insight into what it is like for him to be an outsider.

After completing a go-around, the leader, Peggy, can ask Salvador whether he feels any different and whether he is interested in exploring separateness from others as a possible theme in his life. He tells Peggy that he does feel lonely in his marriage. She might then suggest a role-playing situation such as this: "Pick out the person here who most reminds you of your wife, and talk to her about what you have been saying to us. Perhaps you could say to her some things you haven't said before." Salvador may say, "I can't do that. No one here reminds me of my wife. I don't see what good this would do."

In dealing with Salvador's hesitancy, Peggy should be aware of how Salvador is affecting her and might ask herself how much investment she has in leading him further than he seems to want to go. She may need to remind herself that Salvador has spent a lifetime not expressing himself. Here again, we advocate joining him in the resistance: "OK, Salvador. No one here is going to make you do anything you don't want to do. I hope that you will tell us what you want when you become aware of it." Or, if Peggy has a hunch that he wants some help, she might say, "Salvador, I have a hunch you might be feeling something right now. If you're willing, I'd like you to go ahead and speak to someone here as if she were your wife. You might become more aware of feelings you haven't looked at if you try doing this."

If Salvador does select a person to "become his wife" he can eventually participate in a role reversal exercise by assuming the role of his wife and saying what he imagines she might want to tell him. By reversing roles with his wife, Salvador can gain significant emotional and cognitive insights into both his own situation and his wife's situation. (See Corey, 2004, chap. 8, for a more detailed treatment of the theory underlying psychodramatic techniques.)

Working with a client like Salvador can be difficult. He can easily become the target of group hostility, but that hostility will probably do nothing more than increase his defensiveness. In this situation, it is necessary for Peggy to exercise vigilance to prevent him from being attacked.

Working with Challenges to Leaders

One of the characteristics of the transition stage is the increased willingness of members to begin to confront the leader. This helps pave the way for progressing into the working stage. Initially, the members may politely let much of what the leader says go by, without much reaction. If members do have negative reactions to the leader early in the group, they frequently keep these reactions to themselves. As the group progresses, members generally show more willingness to express some of the things they have been thinking and internally rehearsing. Indeed, the challenge to leadership can free up members to feel safe enough to begin to confront one another more readily.

How this challenge is dealt with is crucial to the future of the group. If leaders are excessively defensive and refuse to acknowledge criticism, they inhibit the members from confronting one another, with a resulting deleterious effect on the level of trust within the group. In essence, such leaders have established a double standard, one set of norms for intermember confrontation and another set for leader confrontation.

Challenges to leaders are rarely without some foundation in reality. Even though there may be symbolic value or an element of transference in such feedback, at this juncture it is best for leaders to take the feedback at face value. Leaders who are too quick to interpret such feedback as projection or transference run the risk of closing off the member and teaching the group to be excessively cautious about confronting. The ultimate goal, of course, is that members learn that their reactions to others can teach them a great deal about themselves, but at this stage they should simply be encouraged to trust their reactions enough to express them. The leader may want to make a mental note to return at some other time to the possible historical context of the feedback.

Leaders can expect to receive some accurate perceptions both of their role as leaders ("When Mary Ellen cried this morning, you seemed to leave her hanging." "Why do you let all this hostility go on?") and of their personal characteristics ("You seem cold and distant!" "You're very authoritarian!"). As a leader, you need not apologize excessively for or defend your behavior, but you do need to explore what members say. Ask questions such as these: "Help me understand better how I may have been cold and distant." "I'd like to get a clearer sense of what felt like an attack to you." "Is there something you wish I had done for Mary Ellen so she wouldn't have been left hanging?" We want to emphasize that in this situation the same rules apply to the leader as to the members. This is an opportunity to model self-disclosure and a genuine willingness to listen to feedback. Leaders should not abdicate their leadership responsibilities by making token disclosures, by insisting that they are "just another member," or by embarking on an endless analysis of their characters.

"Why do we always have to focus on the negative?" Roz brings up the issue of her impatience with the group co-leaders, whom she sees as expecting the members to come up with serious problems all the time. She continues by saying: "We always have to have some problem to talk about. There's so much focus on pain in here. I don't see what stops us from talking about some positive things. I get depressed every time I leave this group, and, besides, I'm tired of listening to everyone's problems. I feel pressured by the leaders to always have something to bring in here."

Before deciding on a technique to use here, the leaders can attempt to discover what Roz means when she says that there is too much focus on the negative. They can ask her to talk more about the pressure she feels from them to have a "problem." They might ask her how the group could be more helpful to her. Here are some possible meanings of her concern over focusing on the negative:

- Roz may have learned to deal with conflict by avoiding it or attempting to smooth things over. When conflict surfaces in the group, she gets uncomfortable and attempts to do what she typically does in everyday life.
- She may have a lot of pain that she is afraid to acknowledge. Having other members talk about their pain triggers her own anxiety, so she'd rather they focus on pleasant topics.
- Perhaps she is afraid of her depression. If she allows herself to feel depressed, she may fear that she will sink so deeply into it that she won't be able to pull herself out. Thus, she would rather talk of positive things that won't lead to depression.
- Roz may have "problem envy" and fear that her own struggles, which seem less pressing than those of the others, won't be welcome.
- She may be afraid of anger. For example, she may have experienced considerable anxiety when another member directed anger at her. Or perhaps simply observing others being angry scares her.
- The leader may indeed be acting somewhat neglectful when serious problems are being dealt with, especially near the end of the meeting.

All these possible meanings involve fears and resistance; techniques for working with them can be adapted from the examples described in the previous section.

If, however, Roz exhibited much feeling when she said that the leaders expected members to come up with problems all the time, they might introduce a technique for working with her projections. One technique is to ask her to become one of the leaders. In taking this role, she can talk to the group and tell them how they should act in the group.

Once Roz's projections and expectations are out in the open, she can work on some of them. For example, one of the leaders might say to her: "In some ways you seem to see us as responsible for the negative feelings in the group, for after all we are the ones who are focusing on these feelings. We could point the group in a different direction and avoid this focus. Do you want to go further with some of the directions you'd rather see this group take and what you'd want us to do differently?" If Roz says yes, she can say what she fears about each member and how she'd rather see that person act so that she would feel comfortable. She might tell Barbara to cheer up and count her blessings instead of dwelling on her misery. She might tell Bob not to get angry because his anger scares her. Again, the leaders can be listening for clues of where to go next with Roz. She may attempt to smooth things over in the group and focus on pleasant matters because she had the role of peacemaker in her family. If she would like to change this behavior, the leaders can then introduce techniques that encourage her to do so.

If trust has been established, the leaders might ask Roz to tell those who have delved into their problems how it was for her to listen to them. She could address these members one at a time and let them know how their work has been affecting her. This could be a catalyst for both her and the others in the group she addresses. They have probably sensed her reactions, and this may be inhibiting them from further discussing their problems. The other members may fear judgment or criticism from her, and this technique will probably bring these reactions to the surface. As a result of talking to those members that she is most tired of hearing from, Roz may uncover some of her dynamics. It could be that she is attempting to avoid facing these very problems. It may also be that these people symbolize someone with whom she has a strained relationship. Again, she could accept the challenge to do some further work if she has decided that it is okay for her to have problems and to work on them in the group.

An alternative strategy for working with Roz is to ask her to complete sentences such as these:

- When people in my life express negative thoughts or feelings, I _______.
- If only the leaders would _______.
- This reminds me of _______.

This sentence-completion technique is designed to expose her reinforcement history and what she has learned from negative experiences throughout her life. The technique can elicit material for further exploration.

"You leaders aren't sharing enough of yourselves." This sort of remark can be a healthy sign in a group because it indicates that members perceive an inequality—namely, that the leaders are different from all the others in the group in that they don't say much about themselves. Not infrequently this complaint is well founded. Examine the degree to which you are willing to make yourself known to the members of your group.

Leaders can abdicate their role if they throw out some tidbit about themselves to placate the group, but we do not advise this. Instead, they might indicate that they are in the group not for their own therapy, as are the members, but to be leaders. They can, of course, share feelings and thoughts concerning the members individually and as a group and acknowledge being touched by personal issues—especially how they feel right now in this confrontation. Leaders will have genuine theoretical differences about the nature and degree of self-disclosure. For example, if they are influenced by the existential approach or person-centered therapy, they are more likely to engage in self-disclosure than if they are psychoanalytically oriented. Leaders need to examine honestly their motivations for discussing their personal issues and ask themselves whether the disclosure serves the members' needs or their own. Leaders also need to be open to evaluating what impact this is having on them and on the group.

Group facilitators can become transparent in many ways without talking about personal problems. Leaders do a disservice to themselves if they have to prove that they, too, are human. It is simply a fact that the group counselor does have a different purpose for being in the group. Leaders make a mistake if they become intimidated by their different role, and it is important that they do not apologize for this difference. But they must explore what the member means by "sharing enough of yourselves." They might ask, "How would it be helpful to you if I told you more about myself?" The tone in which they respond to members who want more disclosure is crucial. Either they can convey nondefensiveness and a willingness to reflect about what is being said, or they can respond in a sharp and critical manner that conveys a sense of superiority. Leaders do not have to give the impression that they have arrived and are now "actualized beings." They can let members know that they are still struggling with issues in their own lives but that they do not highlight these issues in the groups they are leading. When group facilitators do engage in self-disclosure, it is important to attend to the members and not to deter them from exploring their own issues. (For a more detailed treatment of self-disclosure and genuineness as key concepts of the person-centered approach to groups, see Corey, 2004, chap. 10.)

Leaders might examine the motives of members who ask them to show more of themselves. Often such a challenge is based on the members' need to relieve their own anxiety or to have some of the pressure taken off. Other times the motive might be to make the leader seem less intimidating.

Some leaders may feel comfortable sharing not only present reactions but old feelings that come to the surface because of someone else's work. This material can be a catalyst for further group work. Leaders should not display these feelings, however, simply because group members want them to. They may find that attuning themselves to their feelings, both those that arise in the present context and those nurtured through reminiscing about their past, is actually their best tool for listening to others.

Other leaders may be less interested in expressing their own feelings as a prerequisite for leading. If the feelings are there or if they come up within the course of a group, they may express them, but they don't feel the need to stir them up. Some leaders also may not be able to switch in and out of their own intense feelings fast enough to keep their primary focus on the client, to be fully with the group member's work rather than their own. If a personal issue interferes with being with the client, leaders may work on it in the group, perhaps only in order to get clear enough to continue work with the client. It is important, however, for leaders to bring into the group any persistent feelings they have that stand in the way of their being able to work with a client. For example, if a leader feels some degree of anger, boredom, or annoyance toward a client, the leader may not immediately share these feelings. However, if these feelings persist and get in the way of working with the client, the leader eventually may need to disclose this so that it does not interfere with the relationship between leader and client. Ideally, this both clears the air and puts the leader's reactions at the service of the client. One of the best ways to teach members about feelings is for the leader to express his or her own feelings.

The main point here is that leaders should not be working on their own material in the group at the expense of the client. Very clear countertransference issues might be best addressed in supervision or personal therapy. Yet leader openness can surely make a contribution to the enhancement of the group process. If a member brings up a fear of being inadequate, leaders can mention similar concerns of their own in a way that encourages the member to go further. But if the whole group stops so that leaders get to talk about their feelings of inadequacy, the purpose of the group has been lost, and the role of the leader is blurred. If leaders are involved in their own growth, as they should be, they will find that most personal matters can be postponed for discussion with their own therapists.

"You leaders aren't very helpful." This challenge can take many forms. Members may say that leaders "don't really care for us," "are against us," "are directing us too much," "aren't directing us enough," "aren't getting us started," "are pushing people too much," "leave people hanging," "focus too much on pain and hurt," "are using this group to fulfill your own needs," "don't really know what you're doing," or "seem to have a lot of hang-ups, so how can you lead us?"

This challenge can be seen as a healthy signal that a group is becoming autonomous. In this situation, defensiveness can do damage. You cannot simply dismiss such confrontations as a stage the group is going through, nor can you too readily assume that you are failing. You might ask the members: "What are you wanting from me that you're not getting?" Or you might say: "Tell me more. What am I doing or not doing that is not helpful?" As members respond, listen and avoid reacting too quickly or in a defensive manner. Once you have taken in what was said, you can then share your reactions about what you heard and how it affected you. In this way you are dealing with your thoughts and feelings as they pertain to what is occurring within the group. At a moment like this, you can model the behavior you hope the group members will learn, including a willingness to explore matters that might trigger a defensive posture.

Here you might ask group members how they would like things to be different, if indeed they would, and then to say whether you, as a leader, are willing to do what the members want and why. For example, members may say that they want you to introduce techniques when they feel stuck or when there are long silences. You might reply that you do not want to take on total responsibility for the direction of the group and that you hope that the members will accept their share of the responsibility for what gets accomplished. This sort of comment allows members to clarify what they want and allows you to discuss your own views openly. In fact, you might respond initially to a challenge by saying what you would like to see going on in the group.

In the responses suggested so far, you are seeking to acknowledge the legitimate parts of the challenge. Of course, you can also explore the possibility of projections. Complaints may be more important for what they say about the members than what they say about the leaders. If you have modeled receptiveness and an ability to handle situations in which you feel defensive, you are in a good position to ask group members to explore the part of themselves that finds fault with others.

"You blew it." Most group leaders, not just the novice, worry at times about making mistakes. In one sense, any input you give as a leader can provide material worth exploring. Regardless of whether members think you are marvelous or a flop, the way they respond can teach them much about themselves. You will function better once you begin to worry less, because you then free up your spontaneity and intuition. For all that, all leaders have moments that qualify as mistakes—interventions they regretted or techniques they would have preferred to use differently. Mistakes occur when leaders impose their own agenda rather than being sufficiently ready to follow and flow with the client.

The most effective way to handle a misdirected technique is to admit the mistake. We've rarely felt that we lost the respect of our clients when we admitted our mistakes. But we have found that troubles multiply if we are unwilling to admit mistakes and try to just forge ahead. It's a perfect opportunity to model making such an admission without undue defensiveness or remorse. Usually, the emotional momentum that may have been dissipated by the inappropriate intervention can be recovered after such an admission. Sometimes it can't, but the issue that was lost may come up again. The important points here are that you should not hide behind your role or assume you must be perfect and that you should not try to cover up a mistake by imposing yet another technique. As long as you are not trying to hide behind your techniques, it may sometimes be productive to create a technique for constructively exploring your group's reaction once you've gone wrong.

Here are some mistakes that we've made as group practitioners:

- We have given instructions that were too elaborate, complicated, or obscure.
- We have been too hasty in introducing a technique when we were not clear enough about what our members were saying or where we wanted to go with them.
- We have not been sufficiently sensitive to a member's resistance to going along with a technique.
- We have pursued too rigidly an outcome we expected a technique to have and have not been sufficiently tuned in to where a participant was leading us.
- Our interjection of humor has been out of tune with a member's seriousness.

- We have timed techniques poorly, usually because we were not sensitive enough to the member's own pace and were too fixed on our own interpretations or hopes concerning the individual.
- We have set up role-playing situations in which we asked people to take parts that we forgot would be painfully inappropriate for them.
- We have introduced techniques for generating material when we were insufficiently attuned to hidden agendas and issues already present in the group.
- We have had techniques and catalysts in mind for a session and have failed to realize we had too much planned or have failed to be sufficiently attuned to the issues and moods our members brought with them.
- After being threatened, we have become defensive and have been less therapeutic than we might have been.
- We have failed to respond in a personal way to a member who deserved a personal reaction.
- We have introduced an icebreaker technique to get things going when there was no need for it because the group was already prepared to work.
- We were impatient with silence.

Concluding Comments

During the transition stage of a group, key tasks for the leader are to continue building trust and cohesion in the group; to continue to invite members to recognize and deal with their fears, anxieties, and hesitations; to be aware of negative reactions and conflict within the group; to point out the value of recognizing and dealing with intermember conflict; to model nondefensive behavior when challenged; to work toward decreasing the dependence of members on the leader and increasing individual responsibility; to encourage members to express persistent feelings about the group; to help members learn how to recognize their ways of avoiding and to teach them ways of challenging their resistances; to teach members directness and effective confrontation; and to enable members to decide on ways in which they are willing to be different in the group.

We conclude this section with some guidelines for effective confrontation. For both members and leaders alike, confrontation is a delicate matter that all too often is handled without sufficient skill and sensitivity. Unless techniques are presented in a caring manner, they are likely to be ineffective in getting participants to recognize and deal with their resistance. One of the functions of a leader is to model constructive confrontation for members and to teach them how to confront one another in an honest and sensitive manner. Here are a few guidelines that you may want to apply to yourself:

- Confrontation is based on the assumption that you care about the person being confronted. This caring is expressed by being respectful. It may be helpful for you to imagine yourself as the recipient of the confrontation you are delivering.

- If you are confronting a person, it is a good idea to make a statement about yourself to let that individual know your purpose in confronting him or her. You might say, "Your opinion matters to me, and I wish you would talk more in this group."
- In confronting others, speak primarily about yourself and how you are affected by what they are doing or saying in the group. It may be more accurate to say "I am having a great deal of difficulty talking to you about this matter" than to say "You are impossible to talk to about this matter." The latter statement is bound to promote defensiveness.
- In confronting people, describe what you see them doing, and avoid labeling them or judging them. It is not helpful to tell a person that he or she talks too much and is a monopolizer. A more effective confrontation is "I want to listen to you and understand you, but I sometimes get lost in your words and don't know what you really want me to hear."
- Confront in a way that encourages others to continue behaving in the way you would like to see them act. Chances are that a person will be put off if you say "You never talk, and it's about time you opened up in here." But they may be helped to express themselves if you say "I really like it when you talk, and I learn a lot from you."
- Be sensitive to the timing of your confrontation. For example, don't confront a member on insufficient participation at a moment when he or she is talking. Instead, reinforce the individual's attempts at making a change.
- Above all, remember that honesty without caring and compassion can be cruel.

Questions and Activities

1. How would you describe the characteristics of groups in their transition stage? What do you see as your main tasks as a leader at this stage?
2. How would you work with a member who rejects all attempts to work through resistance? How would your strategy be influenced by whether the group was voluntary or involuntary?
3. Imagine you are a member of a group. What behaviors of yours would constitute resistance? In what specific ways would you resist? What techniques would be especially effective or ineffective in encouraging you to work through your resistance?
4. What criteria can you use to determine whether a group member whom you consider difficult is actually behaving counterproductively in the group or whether this member is evoking some of your unresolved personal issues?
5. What general guidelines can you come up with for dealing effectively with group members who exhibit problematic behaviors?
6. A group member uses attention-getting behavior whenever the focus is not on him for any length of time, and when attention does center on him, he talks at length, boring or irritating others in the group. Can you think of any techniques for such a situation?

7. Fred is typically sarcastic and hostile. He stops the work of others with his indirect remarks. You sense that the trust level is being lowered by his manner of venting his anger. How would you handle this situation? What might you do about the other members' reactions to him?
8. Sandy typically tells others how they should be, and she is quick to provide solutions to their problems. While aborting their work, she also keeps the focus off herself. Can you think of any techniques that you might use in this situation?
9. Imagine how group members might become hostile toward Salvador when he says that he can't identify with anyone in the group. Describe some possible techniques for working with this situation. If Salvador made his remarks at a preliminary session, would you be likely to include him in or exclude him from the group? Why?
10. Your group members say they are stuck and getting nowhere. What are your thoughts about their complaint and about your responsibility for getting them moving?
11. Jill comments on not feeling safe in her group. If you were a member in a group, what would it require to make you feel safe in it? How might a leader best work with you on this topic?
12. Look over the list of difficult members in this chapter and think of others whom you might find difficult. Which one pattern of problem behavior do you think you would have the most trouble with? Speculate about the personal dynamics that might be involved in your reactions to this behavior.
13. Some conflicts and struggles for power are inevitable in a group. How do you think techniques can be used in working with conflict? Do you believe conflict can have therapeutic value in a group? Explain.
14. At the fifth meeting, a member who has been relatively silent finally confronts you with his lack of trust in your leadership ability. How might you deal with this challenge?
15. In a group you are leading, a considerable amount of intermember conflict is expressed in several sessions. Finally, a timid and quiet man asks, "Why are you allowing all this conflict and bickering to take place? What good is all of this doing anybody?" What might you say, and where might you be inclined to go from there?
16. What techniques can you think of to get members to see connections between the sessions? How might you help them work outside the group and bring their results back to a following session?
17. There are many meanings underlying most forms of resistance. How could you facilitate a member's exploration of the meaning of some defensive behavior that you might find annoying?
18. Consider the pattern of behavior you typically model as a group leader. What kind of group might you have if all of the members in it displayed the behavior that you model?
19. What are some of the ways in which you would explore a client's cultural background as a way of understanding his or her difficult behavior?

20. How would you go about evaluating your own effectiveness as a leader, especially when your group seemed to be experiencing rough times? How would you assess your degree of responsibility as well as the members' responsibility if the group seemed stuck?

Guide to Using *Groups in Action: Evolution and Challenges* DVD and Workbook

First Program: *Evolution of a Group*

1. *Characteristics of the transition stage.* The transition stage is often characterized by conflict. What characteristics unfold in the group during the transition stage? What evidence do you see of dealing with anxiety, resistance, and conflict?
2. *Dealing with members who are difficult.* What are some difficult member behaviors that you notice in the group in the first program?
3. *Dealing with conflict.* Although conflict often occurs during the transition stage, it can erupt during the initial group session. In the DVD group, conflict occurs during both the initial and the ending stages. What did you learn about how to deal with conflict regardless of when it occurs? What are the possible consequences of ignoring conflict or dealing with it ineffectively?
4. *Exploring common fears and resistance.* The text deals with themes pertaining to common fears of group members. Various members of the DVD group also express fears, including these:

   - "I'm afraid that people will judge me."
   - "If I express my hurt, my fear is that people won't want to listen to me."
   - "I'm afraid that I won't fit in this group. I feel like a kid in here."

   What did you learn from the DVD program about what is helpful in exploring fears such as these? What lessons can you learn about how to close a particular group session? How do the co-leaders encourage members to put words to what they experienced in a given group session?
5. *Challenges during the transition stage.* During the transition phase, the anxiety in a group is high because members are beginning to risk letting themselves be known on a deeper level. We ask members to talk more about whatever fears or reservations they may be experiencing. We see our task as intervening in a way that makes the room safer and providing a climate whereby members can talk about their hesitations. After viewing the first program, what is the importance of carefully working with whatever members bring to a group regarding their fears and reservations? How is this transitional work essential if you hope to help a group move to a deeper level of interpersonal interaction? What are you learning about the leader's task during this crucial stage in a group?

CHAPTER SIX

Techniques for the Working Stage

Introduction

In this chapter we concentrate on some typical remarks members make during the working stage of a group. Although some of these remarks are rather common, they won't necessarily arise in every group, nor will they always seem important. Removed from their context, these remarks by clients may not strike a counselor as profound or promising. Yet given the context of work in progress with a group member, they can be excellent springboards for introducing techniques to pursue a leader's hunch.

The statements that a leader picks out often reflect the leader's energy and interests as well as the client's. When we work with a statement, we do not know in advance exactly where it will lead. As often as not, an intervention may develop in an unanticipated direction. In this chapter on the working stage, we are assuming that the leader knows the client well enough to have a good hunch about the outcome of the work. The objective is to find ways of bringing issues and feelings into focus, and the statements we discuss here have the promise of helping achieve this objective.

We want to emphasize again that leaders must be willing to abandon a technique and follow whatever material seems to be immediate. We introduce techniques, but clients let us know what direction to pursue. When a group member is already showing some emotion, it is distracting to spend a great deal of time setting up a technique. The sensitivity and spontaneity of a good leader is acquired through practice and supervision, and we encourage you to pursue such opportunities. We rarely enter a group with a set idea of the techniques we are going to use. Instead, we develop these techniques during the session, basing them on promising clues and introducing them in such a way as to lead a client into the exercise gracefully and quickly.

An underlying rationale for most of the interventions we suggest is that it is not the leader's role to make people feel good or to solve their problems. People must work out for themselves the solutions to the problems they face. However, leaders can provide a setting in which members, through intensifying their thoughts and feelings and sorting them out, can make more informed choices. The leader can provide the structure that enables members to pursue different options in their struggles. This is the main task of the working stage.

Characteristics of the Working Stage

During the working stage, we focus on linking members by looking for and pursuing common themes within the group. Leaders should be alert to opportunities for bringing other group members into the work of an individual client. Often part of the reason for picking a specific statement to use in devising a technique is that it seems a promising avenue for including other group members. One of the signs that a group has reached the working stage is the members' ability to spontaneously bring themselves into one another's work. A working group involves a level of cohesion that allows for two or more individuals to work simultaneously on common issues, as opposed to members' taking turns by doing their individual work in a group setting.

A characteristic of the working stage is that participants are usually, although not always, eager to initiate work or bring up themes they want to explore. They do not come to the group saying, "Well, I don't know what I want to talk about tonight; I thought I'd go with whatever comes up for me." Being open to dealing with emerging reactions is fine, for it can lead to some productive work, but the person who says "I don't know what I want from this session" is often reflecting a passive stance. Many members in a working group will be clear about what they want and will ask for group time. The leader may begin a session with a simple "Who wants to work?" and find that several members declare that they want some time.

This stage is also characterized by a here-and-now focus. A sign of a productive group is that members have learned to talk about what they are currently feeling and doing. Hence, typically their work has a direct quality rather than a detached storytelling style. Even though members may be exploring problems they have with people outside of the group, they do their work by dealing with their present feelings and thoughts about these problems. They also bring problems from their past into the present by working symbolically with significant people in their lives as if those people were present in the room. While an individual is working on outside issues, the leader can also pay attention to what is occurring with other members. By this time, members typically are affected by each other's work and are willing to acknowledge this. The group has progressed beyond politely waiting until an individual's work is finished. Members have learned that they can enhance another's work by spontaneously expressing ways in which they are identifying with that person's struggle.

Members are also willing to have direct and meaningful interactions with one another, including confrontations. Conflict in the group is recognized, and members have learned that they need not run away from it. Members are not likely to suppress their feelings of conflict with one another simply because this difficulty is not always immediately resolved. This behavior is quite different from what many of them have learned in their outside lives, where they have demonstrated an "allergic reaction" to sticking with interpersonal conflicts until they are worked through. For instance, assume that Amber says to Fritz, "I wish you weren't in the group, because I don't like you." This comment certainly needs to be addressed. Amber would be asked to give her reactions more directly to Fritz and what led up to the conclusions she has formulated about him. She would be challenged to deal with her reactions to him, and he would be given a chance to deal with her, which could open up productive material for both of them. A working group reflects a commitment of people to stay with others through difficult times until all sides have a chance to be given expression. Conflict is not ignored but in fact becomes the focus for work. How people work through their conflicts in the group situation (or how they avoid doing so) offers many lessons for participants about the sources of their interpersonal problems.

Other characteristics differentiate the working stage from the initial and the transition stages. Members more readily identify their goals and concerns, and they have learned to take responsibility for them. They are less confused about what the group and the leaders expect of them. Most of the participants feel included in the group, or if some do not, they can talk about it in the group. Participants trust the leader's interpretations and suggestions and are less cautious about going along with proposed techniques. Communication in the group is characterized by a free give and take among the members and a tendency for them to engage in direct exchanges rather than communicating by way of the leader. The individual members listen to one another and do productive work together.

Members trust themselves more and are more ready to speak their minds, to experiment with different behaviors, and to push themselves to explore personal issues that they find frightening. They are hopeful about the potential for meaningful gain from their participation, and they take more responsibility not only for what goes on within the group but also for carrying what they are learning into their outside lives. They commonly engage in work involving the expression of emotion and are not as frightened by it because they have had a chance to see such emotions expressed in constructive ways. They are less concerned about whether they will be accepted for what they say, having seen the group accept people who have shared difficult aspects of themselves. Self-disclosure is the norm and is seen as appropriate. The members are willing to try to integrate thinking, feeling, and behaving in their everyday life. Issues of transference between members and the leader come out in the open more readily, and members are used to seeing what this transference can teach them about their past and present experiences outside the group. Not all confrontations will be successful in the working stage, but it is more likely that they will be effective.

Intermember exchanges during the working stage are characterized by giving and receiving honest, direct, caring, and useful feedback. Members tend to be more trusting of the suggestions they receive, for they now know that people who give them feedback are also willing to receive it.

Group cohesion increases during the working phase. The members have worked together to develop a trusting community, and they respect and care for one another. This sense of community encourages members to explore themselves on a deeper level than is typically true in the beginning stages of the group. The group has earned a level of cohesion through the process of sharing pain, the pain that unites them in their common human experience of struggling. Members who are different in many respects have also found common ground that enables them to take significant risks with one another.

This cohesion is not a static entity, however, and like trust, it can ebb and flow. After a very intense session in which intense work has been done, members are sometimes frightened by the feelings that have been generated.

They may temporarily become more distant, and it may look as though the level of cohesion is waning.

Having said all of this, we also want to point out that the working stage is not always characterized by catharsis and a deeper exploration of issues. In some groups there can be an absence of intense emotions, yet the group still functions well and achieves its goals. For example, in task groups, psychoeducational groups, guidance groups, structured groups, and theme-oriented groups, the participants can be talking honestly, there can be a sense of immediacy, and there can be meaningful interchanges. These group members may show a willingness to cooperate in working on a common agenda, and they may be very committed to the group. They may also demonstrate a willingness to express their differences openly and to struggle with one another to get to the place they would like to reach as a group. In some working groups there may never be a high level of emotional intensity, yet there can still be an honest exchange between members. The interactions may focus on more subtle and seemingly less intensely personal issues, but the key point is that the group is characterized by a willingness to work through material rather than shelving issues.

Not all groups reach the stage that we are describing, but that does not necessarily mean that the leader is ineffective. Other factors can keep the group from going beyond the initial stage. Variable membership in a group can inhibit attaining the working stage, particularly if there is no stable core of members willing to work. Some populations may simply never be ready for the level of intensity we have described. For groups to develop emotional intensity, a therapeutic climate must have been established earlier that makes it possible to engage in a deeper level of risking and personal sharing. Some groups have not established a safe climate, because the members have not yet committed themselves to the demanding work required of a productive group. For example, the participants may be mandated through the courts and may not be willing members. Even so, members have the opportunity to learn much about themselves at all stages of a group.

If the members did not work through the initial stage effectively, the working stage may never be reached. The members may be unwilling to give of themselves beyond what is necessary for superficial encounters. They may have collectively decided to stop at a safe and supportive level of interaction rather than to challenge one another, much as some married couples do. Early interchanges between members and the leader or among the members may have been characterized by harsh and uncaring words or actions. The resulting climate does not encourage members to take the risks necessary to move to a deeper level of interaction. The group may see itself as a problem-solving group. This orientation replaces self-exploration, for as soon as a member raises a problem the other members look for immediate solutions. For these reasons and others, some groups never progress into what we describe as the working stage.

When a group does get to the working stage, it doesn't progress as neatly and tidily as our characterization may suggest. Earlier themes of trust, nonconstructive conflict, and reluctance to participate surface again and again. As we have said, trust is a process, not a state. As the group faces new challenges, deeper levels of trust have to be earned. Also, considerable conflict may be resolved in the initial stage, but new conflicts emerge and must be faced. In a sense, a group is like any intimate relationship: it is not static, and perfection is never reached.

Working with Emerging Themes

In this section we present a variety of themes that might emerge in a working group. Our intention is to give some sense of the struggles that individuals bring to the sessions and to demonstrate possible techniques in helping members explore their concerns in more depth. As will become evident, some of the following statements sound like ones that could be made during the transition period in a group's development. In the working stage, however, the members show a willingness to go beyond the point at which they have typically stopped because of anxiety. Their commitment to work often has the effect of triggering other members, which can easily lead to the development of common themes that unite the group.

"I'm confused and don't know what to do." A statement expressing confusion can have many different explanations. The use of a technique is not dictated just by a member's statement, but it also includes how the leader views the member's participation in the group and how all of this is processed.

When Bettina says "I'm confused," the leader understands that she is stuck and unable to proceed. The leader may theorize that there is something that Bettina does not want to know or to take a stand on. That information is not shared with her, but the leader devises a technique to assist her in exploring that possibility. Directly confronting Bettina would just entrench the resistance. Instead, the leader asks Bettina, "What do you want to do now?" or "What do you want to say now?" Alternatively, the leader might say, "Do whatever you want to do." In agreeing with her and in a sense handing the direction of the work over to her, the leader leaves her with no one to resist. This technique bypasses resistance and allows her to lead the way.

Depending on the leader's relationship with Bettina, he might say to her: "Pretend you weren't confused. What would you be saying now if you knew what you wanted?" A related technique consists of asking her to act for a week as if she were not confused. She can be given the homework assignment to assume that she is clear and confident. If she responds with: "This sounds like a good assignment, and I'm willing to give it a try, but I'm afraid I'll feel even more confused in spite of trying to convince myself that I'm clear. Then what do I do?" The leader could respond with: "Well, are you willing to press on, even if you're confused—and maybe try to assure yourself that you do know what you want?" This is very much like the Adlerian reorientation technique that encourages members to act *as if* they were the persons they wanted to be. Members are asked to "catch themselves" in the process of repeating old patterns that lead to ineffective behavior, such as being confused. (For a more detailed discussion of the rationale of the "as if" technique, see Corey, 2004, chap. 7.)

Another strategy would be to ask Bettina to make an alliance with someone in the group and to call that person to report on how this assignment is going. All these techniques put increased responsibility on her to do something cognitively and behaviorally outside of the group meetings to move beyond the place where she typically gets stuck. Of course, she can bring back to the following session a report of what she learned by carrying out this assignment. This would be an example of a technique based on the behavioral approach to group counseling (see Corey, 2004, chap. 13.)

"I'm afraid to get close to people." When a member (Carl) makes this statement, the leader can begin by asking him whether he wants to explore the issue of closeness. Does Carl want to get close? Is it all right with him if he doesn't? Whom does he want to get close to in his life right now? Sometimes it is not clear how genuinely people are involved with issues they introduce. By asking Carl these questions, the leader can allow him to focus on whether this issue is pressing for him or whether he is getting what he wants as things are now.

If, as Carl talks, the leader senses that this is a significant topic for him but that he is not expressing much affect, she can ask him to talk about the closeness he feels is missing between him and others in the group. Any of these questions could enable him to explore his fear of intimacy within the here-and-now context of the group: "Who might you want to get closer to in here? And what has stopped you so far?" "How close do you think that people in here feel to you? And what might you be doing to either draw people toward you or push them away from you?" "What are some things that you tell yourself when you imagine yourself developing intimacy with us?" "Is there anything you want to say to anyone in here that you've thought about but haven't said?" This technique brings the rest of the group into Carl's work and provides an opportunity for feedback from others about whether he behaves in ways that keep him from having much intimacy with them. It also picks up on his use of the word *afraid* and gives him an opportunity to discuss what the fears might be.

Assume that Carl's fears of closeness stem from parental injunctions, or messages (transactional analysis), and tacit communications such as "Don't get close" or "Be careful who you talk to." In this case, the leader can pursue the topic by asking questions such as these: "What specifically did you hear from your parents or learn nonverbally?" "Who in your life modeled keeping distance?" Next, Carl can pretend he is that person and talk to the members about why they should not get close to anyone. What would this person—perhaps his father—say about his getting close to each member of this group? And what would he want to say in reply to his father? Through this technique Carl can come to understand how he carries out these parental injunctions by being the way he has been in the group. The leader can continue by getting him to look at early decisions he made, such as "If I don't get close, I won't be hurt" or "I'm not going to be hurt again by being abandoned." The leader can then return to how Carl currently keeps himself from closeness in the group and in everyday life. The leader's aim with this intervention is to assist Carl in seeing ways he keeps an old fear of closeness present in his life. Carl is aware that distance is now causing him pain. With this insight, it is up to Carl to determine if he wants to make any changes from these early decisions. (For a more complete discussion of the key concepts of injunctions, early decisions, and redecisions, see Corey, 2004, chap. 12.)

"This isn't the real world." Cheryl brings up a problem that she wants to explore in the group. She doubts whether she can apply what she experiences in the group to her life at work and at home. She feels free to disclose her reactions in the group, for she is supported in doing so. She finds the support that she receives from the group very helpful and she cannot imagine that kind of support at home. It is important for group leaders to respect members' hesitancy to be too outspoken at work or home. Therefore, it is the leader's and members' job to assist Cheryl in determining what she can say both at work and at home without dire consequences. Her basic task is to learn what is appropriate disclosure and how to make such disclosures without making others defensive.

The leader asks Cheryl to describe a particularly difficult situation and to say what she'd like to change in it. She says that she doesn't like the way she responds to her co-workers in the office. She experiences herself as extremely careful of what she says to them lest she hurt their feelings or offend them. She constantly censors what she is about to say and attempts to figure out what her co-workers want to hear. She would like to feel free to tell these people what's on her mind. After sketching the situation, Cheryl can select several "co-workers" from the group, describe an incident in the office, and tell how she typically would act in this situation. Then, she can tell each of the co-workers in the group things she would not normally say, and say aloud what she is thinking and telling herself as she is talking with each of them.

This intervention might uncover how she stops herself from being more forthright. She may be seeking approval from a co-worker. Or she may be suppressing her anger over the way she feels treated by that person. She may be intimidated by another's sarcasm and put-downs. The leader can eventually have her focus on one of the co-workers and say more of what she typically censors out. She can at least be encouraged to tell this person how she is feeling in the person's presence. After the role playing, both the members and the leader can provide feedback to Cheryl by telling her how they might feel if they were her co-worker. How willing would they be to listen to her? How were they affected by her? In short, she can learn how to confront others without increasing their defensiveness. The specific feedback after role playing is helpful to members like Cheryl who may not be aware of how their style of disclosure puts others off. When members role-play in this kind of situation, we observe that they often find ways to talk that are much more respectful and effective.

The leader can use the group process itself to point out to the members how they moved from fear and hesitancy toward being able to say things to each other by expressing difficult reactions. As members become open and trusting in the group, they can begin to take risks selectively with people on the outside. The key word is *selectively.* Cheryl may be setting herself up for failure if she attempts to open up with everyone she knows. She needs to decide how important a given relationship is to her. She may well decide, for example, not to tell her boss everything she thinks, for she might indeed put her job in jeopardy by doing so. It is therapeutic for her to say what she typically keeps bottled up inside of her in the supportive atmosphere of the group, but it may be unwise for her to do the same at work. However, she can still recognize within herself what she is feeling, and she does not have to repress those feelings even though she keeps them to herself. From this experience, she can also learn to find someone with whom she can talk about reactions that she chooses not to express to her boss.

We frequently discuss with members the potential consequences if they said in their everyday life what they sometimes say in role-playing situations in the group. We attempt to teach people how they may not get the results they want if they confront others too directly at work. In a case such as Cheryl's, we would help her examine the consequences that might follow if she decided to confront people in her life. We don't tell her not to confront, but we do help her assess the risks involved and help her decide what she most wants to say and what she might not want to say to others. Through her work in the group, she may discover that some of her reactions toward her boss are the result of transference. Her boss may be getting more of her reactions than he or she deserves. Part of the group process involves providing members with skills that will lead to bridging the gap between the group and the real world.

"I'm afraid I might never stop crying." Although many people in the group have taken significant risks and allowed themselves to begin a process of healing, a few members have kept themselves in check and consistently dealt with their problems in a more cognitive manner. Priscilla is aware that she is preventing herself from experiencing the depth of her feelings. She admits that she withholds herself emotionally much of the time, both in her life and in this group. When the leader explores this with her, Priscilla says she is afraid that if she started to cry she might never stop. The leader might ask: "What have you observed in here when members have expressed their emotions and cried?"

The leader can ask Priscilla whether she wants to change the manner in which she deals with her emotions. She might say, "I would like to be more like Selena who is able to express her emotion and at this moment still looks very emotional from work she has just completed." If she agrees, the leader can have Priscilla sit in front of Selena, and talk to her about some of the things she holds back, perhaps even in this group. The emotion still evident in Selena's face may serve as a catalyst for evoking feeling in Priscilla.

Or the leader can ask Priscilla to tell Selena how she is affected by Selena's tears. Priscilla may get through her resistance to crying by talking to Selena about her reaction. During this exercise, the leader might suggest any or all of these sentences for Priscilla to complete as she continues her contact with Selena:

- Selena, when you cried I _______.
- If I were to cry like that, I would _______.
- If I were to cry, I would cry about _______.
- One reason I can't cry is _______.
- Tears don't do any good because _______.
- The people in my life who cried were _______.
- The people in my life who didn't cry were _______.

A series of such sentence-completion suggestions can provide a powerful collaboration between the leader and the member that often spontaneously produces important opportunities for insight. The leader can take cues for further work from Priscilla's replies. Selena is encouraged to respond by saying what it was like for her as Priscilla talked to her. Finally, to connect others in the group to this work, they can be asked to express to either Priscilla or Selena how they were affected by the interaction.

Although typically group members supply the material with which they want to work (as in the case of Bettina and her confusion), leaders may sometimes have a hunch that something else is going on that is not being addressed. Suppose Priscilla still feels stuck. She is sitting before Selena and seems to have no idea what to say. The leader could say to her: "Priscilla, I wonder whether there has ever been a person in your life over whom you needed to cry, yet you didn't allow yourself to?" The leader formulates a broad question in which almost anyone could find something to pursue. The leader's hunch might be that Priscilla is still mourning the death of someone important to her and that her grief contributes to her depressive style. But mentioning death here is too specific and threatening. Instead, the leader gives Priscilla an opportunity and leaves her enough room to pull back.

It might be worth noting that crying has cultural and gender implications. We do not subscribe to the notion that people must cry, nor is it our agenda to get people to cry. However, if members declare that they have a problem with not being able to cry, we explore this with them. If crying is not a problem for them, then it is not a problem for us. Leaders need to be sensitive to group pressure for a member to cry. Group members need to be challenged on their need to see a particular member express deep emotion and cry.

"I'm afraid I'll lose control." Dave, a member of a group composed of relatively well-functioning people, expresses a fear of losing control. As we noted in Chapter 5, it is essential that the leader explore with Dave what he means by "out of control." Leaders and members may know what "out of control" means to them, but at this point, they do not know what it means to Dave. The leader can get him to work with the paradoxical idea that people gain control in their emotional lives when they become willing to lose control, when they give up rigid fears about what they would be like if they did not keep their emotions in check all the time. In doing such work, however, Dave may become so fascinated with acting like an out of control person that the leader is concerned. At this point it may be appropriate for the leader to say something like this: "You know, Dave, I see you working very hard at proving that you could go out of control. So in spite of the fact that I generally encourage people here to be unrestrained in their expression of feeling, I think maybe you could really frighten yourself if you insisted on it. It might be more productive for you to work on not overwhelming yourself!" With this intervention the leader is attempting to get Dave to see that he indeed is contributing to his own frenzy by all the things he is telling himself. It is likely that Dave is afraid he will "go crazy" if he loses control. The leader hopes that she can prevent him from overwhelming himself by taking in too much all at one time. Her intervention is geared to slowing him down and helping him become more centered.

In more normal circumstances, the leader might start out by asking Dave a question: "I wonder where you got the idea that you might 'lose control,' and I wonder what that expression might mean to you?" He may say that there is a history of mental illness in his family. Or he may have been told that expressing anger could make people lose all control. We might ask him: "What does losing control look like, Dave? What does it mean to you?" Dave may say, "I think I would just sit here in a stupor and not interact with anyone." Another member may reply, "It seems to me, Dave, that this is pretty much what you've been doing in this group." The point here is both to acknowledge Dave's concern and to provide a vehicle for confronting it.

Sometimes a group will be ready to work in a more playful way with a theme like the one Dave just introduced. For example, if the circumstances seemed just right, the leader might invite Dave and other members who have expressed the same concern to stage a demonstration of how they think they might behave if they lost control. Through a humorous interaction, some members may recognize that they may spook themselves unnecessarily with the fear of going crazy they associate with losing control. At the same time, the different fantasies of losing control might provide very valuable information about those who participated in this exercise.

Leaders should keep several points in mind in connection with these examples. First, all counselors and group leaders should think through their own theoretical positions about members' fears of losing control and mental illness regardless of whether they work with institutionalized people or relatively well-functioning clients. Our own perspective is that what appears to be "crazy behavior" is at times a way of acting that a client chooses for the purposes of psychological survival. We agree with the assumption of reality therapy that this behavior is often a choice that represents an individual's best attempt to deal with a painful life situation. However, we acknowledge that such behavior is not always a choice, and not all readers will share our theoretical convictions.

Second, leaders who are frightened by their own potential for bizarre behavior can easily reinforce the fears of a client working on this problem and of the rest of the group. Those leaders who are uncertain about their own psychological stability would have a difficult time working with the fears others have of losing control or of acting in crazy ways.

Third, counselors should be cautious in urging clients to go further than they are willing to go themselves. Counselors should not encourage clients to travel a path that they themselves have not walked. What is perhaps most frightening to an inexperienced leader conducting a group composed of presumably relatively well-functioning individuals is to find that someone's behavior is fragmented to a degree that the leader finds unsettling. Experienced leaders who have worked with people like Dave are less inclined to be afraid of clients losing control or acting "crazy." This trust in members is an asset to the work clients are willing and able to do. Among the fears that typically haunt a group, the fear of losing control (of going crazy) is one of the biggest. Here, as elsewhere, the leaders' biggest concern should be for those fears that clients are afraid to express, and leaders can help make the group a place where clients can express and examine those fears.

Fourth, a word of caution. We cannot always know where our techniques are going to lead. It is possible that Dave might start to behave in some bizarre manner. Sometimes the group leader will elect to deescalate the intensity of the work. Then we might urge Dave to keep his eyes open and maintain connection with people in the room by either sitting next to them or talking to them rather than becoming more immersed in his own internal struggles.

Fifth, when a member has done something in the group that he or she regards as weird or bizarre, it is important for the leader to follow up by establishing contact between that member and the group. If this is not done, the person who expressed fears of losing control is likely to withdraw because of embarrassment and concern over what others might be thinking. Invariably, in these situations we do everything we can to encourage members to talk about what they are telling themselves, including how they think others are judging them. Our techniques are aimed at helping them make contact with others in the room by talking about their feelings of embarrassment or their ambivalence. By doing so, they are more apt to stay present and deal with whatever is going on with them.

Working with Intense Emotions in All Members Simultaneously

In this section we describe how a number of members are sometimes triggered by one another's work and become emotionally involved simultaneously. This can occur when clients allow themselves to reexperience painful memories associated with certain life events. At times, they may feel they will lose control. Such emotional energy can be, depending on the group, productive and positive. This is not a usual phenomenon in most groups, but this can never be excluded as a possibility for any group. Members will often trigger each other simultaneously and express a great deal of emotion. If a leader does not know what to do, harm can occur. This phenomenon should not be used as an index to measure a working group. The absence of this phenomenon does not signify that the group is unproductive.

The alert leader can be sensitive to this development by staying attuned not only to the person working but also to others in the group; co-leaders are an asset here. One technique for calming things down is simply to bring the focus back to just one person: "There seems to be a lot of strong emotion in this room. Maybe we could stay with Charlie and what he's dealing with." An alternative direction would be to look for ways to link the work of several members. If you sense that it would be valuable for more than one member to be expressing feelings at the same time, you can invite several people to sit in the center of the group facing one another and share their feelings. Others may be added to this inner working circle either at their own initiative or with your prompting. You need to have sufficient trust in this process to allow it to take its own course. Do not be so concerned with keeping the focus on the person who had been working that you short-circuit the emergence of this phenomenon. Make a mental note to come back to the person who had been in the spotlight when there is an opportunity later.

Once many people have begun expressing their emotions, you have to make a quick decision about which member to work with. You may want to move near or next to a person who is crying. At the same time you must glance about the room to keep track of what is going on elsewhere. At this point all the participants are potential resources for one another and can work constructively together. You may, with a word or gesture, pair people up and have them explore together what they are feeling or offer each other comfort and support. The woman who typically soothes another's pain and never expresses her own is now crying. The man who fears being incapable of loving others may cry silently as he lets himself be with and comfort another member.

For various reasons, you may decide that some members are getting lost in their emotionality. The procedures ordinarily used to intensify emotional expression can be reversed to help a person gain distance and perspective. Having members talk symbolically to a significant person intensifies emotions; talking about the emotion and what they may be learning deintensifies the situation. To deintensify the expression of a member, you might say: "Your mother isn't really here right now. Talk to me about the feelings you have just been expressing and about what you want to learn from this work."

These catharses do not tend to last very long, but it is important that the experience be processed by the group. Check in with the person whose work provided the catalyst to see if he or she needs to finish up, and encourage both those who were clearly involved and those more on the sidelines to put words to their experiences. Help to solidify the learning that should be apparent—that people can allow themselves a period of intense emotional release and be left sane, intact, and peaceful. Although catharsis often results in a healing process, it is important to assist members in formulating insights based on an emotional release. Insight is the cognitive shift that connects awareness of the various emotional experiences with some meaningful narrative. Insight adds a degree of understanding to the catharsis. Catharsis and insight are key concepts of psychodrama (see Corey, 2004, chap. 8).

The material that people express during such cathartic sessions can be important and profound, but it is easy to forget what one was thinking, feeling, and saying. Therefore, as soon as is feasible, ask all members to recall aloud the specifics of what they were experiencing and focus on the insights and feelings they want to remember and learn from.

Working with Dreams

"I had a dream." Patty reports a portion of a dream that she would like to explore. Here are some ideas for working with her. She can report the dream in the present tense, as if it were taking place now. If she can't remember part of the dream, she can invent the missing part, or "dream it up." As she presents the dream, the leader pays attention to her voice, her level of energy, her body posture, and the parts she seems to gloss over as unimportant. At the end of her report, she can say how she felt on awakening, how she felt during the dream, and how she felt while reporting her dream. She can tell what she learned from the dream or how it might tie in with what is going on in her daily life. In short, the leader can try to get an initial sense of what she might think the dream means. To work on the dream in more detail, Patty can assign different parts of it (persons or things) to various members of the group and coach the members on what they might say in those roles. She can tell each person why she picked him or her for the part and why that member was well suited for it. She can also be each part of the dream herself and carry on a dialogue with the other parts. If she was walking toward a door in her dream, she can be the door and talk to Patty and then be Patty and talk to the door. If props are available in the room, Patty can have a dialogue with an actual door. She can also construct a different ending for her dream. Then she or others in the group can act this new ending out. This intervention with Patty illustrates the Gestalt approach to dream work (see Corey, 2004, chap. 11). The Gestalt approach does not interpret and analyze dreams. Instead, the intent is to bring the dream back to life, to re-create it, and to relive it as if it were happening now.

Another technique for working on Patty's dream in detail is to invent sentence completions from the key phrases or concepts in the dream. For example, she can start by saying "If I were a door I would _______." Or, if she used the word *scared* in reporting the dream, she can complete several versions of the sentence, "What scares me most in my life right now is _______."

To involve other members more directly, the leader can ask those who seem especially interested to talk about Patty's dream as if it were their own and to act out various parts. Or members can free-associate to what they regard as interesting symbols in the dream. The group members can also argue over and decide which parts of the dream they want to act out according to their own fantasies. The point here is not for them to interpret for Patty but to use her dream as a tool for looking at themselves.

Techniques for working with dreams can be modified or abandoned as other issues or reactions from others in the group begin to surface. Involving other members enables the leader to use Patty's dream to work with her and others in the group simultaneously. In addition, simply allowing the client to report a dream without elaborate attempts at interpretation is valuable. There may be little necessity for the use of techniques at all.

"I had a dream about the group." Sometimes a member reports a dream that involves the group. Melissa reports such a dream on the third group meeting: "I am in the back of a big tractor with Brendon (the group leader) driving it. The tractor has no trailer attached, just the cab. We are driving through this small town when, suddenly, faceless people stop our cab and start beating on the windows. I cry out to Brendon 'Do something.' and he says 'Don't worry, there's no danger.' I look around and these faceless people seem to be all over the place, attacking people in the town. But then I notice that nobody seems to get hurt and no harm seems to have been done." Melissa can increase her awareness by exploring her dream through the use of Gestalt therapy methods that involve her "becoming" all the parts of her dream (see Corey, 2004, chap. 11).

She can begin by speaking *as Melissa:* "I'm Melissa. I'm in this big tractor with Brendon driving. I feel very safe and happy in here with him driving. I'm going to curl up in the sleeping compartment of this tractor and go to sleep." *As Brendon:* "I'm Brendon. I know what I'm doing. I know where to take this rig, and I feel good about what I'm doing." *As the tractor:* "I'm a great big tractor. I'm strong. I'm made of steel, and I command respect wherever I go. I haul heavy burdens for long periods, and I provide safety to those who ride in my cab." *As the faceless people:* "We are faceless people. We terrify others. They cringe and try to hide from us, and they think we're going to beat them up and kill them." *As Melissa to Brendon:* "Do something. You're the driver. You're supposed to help me. I trusted you, and yet here you are doing nothing to protect us." *As Brendon to Melissa:* "Don't worry. Be patient. You'll see that no harm comes to anybody. You're safe in here even though it looks dangerous."

Melissa obviously is struggling with trust, both of Brendon's leading and of the group members. The next step is to have her tell the "faceless people" in the group how she sees them as dangerous and attacking. She can also tell Brendon how he is not protecting her.

Don't worry too much about what a dream "really means." Instead, look for what meaning can be created with the help of dream materials. In that spirit, it is often useful to treat a dream "as if" it were about the group rather than implying that this is in fact what the dream is all about.

For example, after an initial and somewhat sluggish check-in by all the members of an ongoing weekly group, Raphael reports this dream: "I was alone, and for some reason I was afraid there was going to be this earthquake. And then there was an earthquake of sorts, except that it wasn't any violent shaking or anything like that. There was just this big chasm that started to appear, and where I was sitting was a piece of land that separated from the land on the other side, and it just drifted farther and farther away."

The leader makes a few efforts to draw out further thoughts from Raphael about this dream, but little seems to come to his mind. Eventually the leader proposes this: "You know, Raphael, I really don't have much of a sense of what's going on in your dream, but it does serve to help me express something that's going on in this group. I thought there was some tension here a couple of weeks ago that wasn't addressed last week, and like the earthquake that never quite happened, I'm thinking there's something that's not happening here tonight." Now Melissa speaks up: "That sure fits for me. I'm feeling as if Janice and I are drifting apart after what we disagreed about a few meetings ago, and now it seems this whole group is afraid of an earthquake." The leader says: "I wonder if the group is willing to acknowledge Raphael's dream as a metaphor for describing what we need to be addressing within this group." Raphael says, "Well, I think we're each going to feel as isolated and alone as I do in this dream if we can't be a bit more honest with each other in this group."

We like working with dreams in our groups and we often use the Gestalt therapy approach in exploring and understanding dreams. Doing so actively involves the members in interpreting their own dreams. It is our contention that the associations members make about their own dreams are more accurate and helpful than a leader's interpretations.

Working with Projections and Other Problems of Self-Awareness

"I can't talk to my parents." In response to Dee's complaint that she cannot talk to her parents, we are likely to begin like this: "Let's see whether we can learn more about what makes you feel this way. I'd like you to pick out two people here who can pretend to be your parents. Don't worry about whether there's any real similarity. All you need are two pairs of eyes to look at as you proceed. Now, talk directly to your symbolic parents, and tell them why you find it hard to talk to them." Dee can start off with the sentence "Mom (Dad), it's hard to talk to you because _______." or "When I try to talk with you, I feel _______." By talking directly to her "parents," Dee mobilizes feelings that she may avoid by merely talking *about* her parents. This gives Dee a chance to practice communicating in a direct and honest way. This technique may lead to exploring the content of what Dee won't talk about with her parents, or it may lead to clarifying the process of that communication and how it is inhibited. Thus it provides her with an opportunity both for practicing what she experiences as difficult and for gaining insight into the nature of the difficulty. This approach rests largely on concepts and techniques of psychodrama, which assumes that exploration is more lively and meaningful if the parents are symbolically brought into the here-and-now group context. Some specific techniques of psychodrama that could be useful here include self-presentation, role reversal, and role rehearsal (see Corey, 2004, chap. 8).

Our request that Dee not worry about any real similarity between her actual parents and the symbolic parents forestalls her from saying that no one in the group is much like her parents. That may be true, but it doesn't provide much to work with. The symbolic parents may turn out to be good substitute parents, and the material they open up can be explored either by her or by the group members who are the parents. Depending on context and hunches, we may want to encourage the parents to respond to Dee. They might let her know how they are affected by the feedback they are getting. Her work could even stimulate feelings in the parents about their own children. In this case, it could be very useful for all involved to continue working in this vein.

Initially, it may be best for Dee to get things out in the open without interruption; after she has had a chance to express herself to her parents, they can respond. But an emotionally productive and relevant scene may emerge from a dialogue between Dee and her parents, especially if she does some coaching or role reversing. Even inappropriate input from one of the parents can be used to advantage. For instance, Dad may do more talking than listening until Dee becomes frustrated enough to say that in real life her father's similar behavior is part of the problem. Almost any material that comes out of such an interaction can be very productive to explore further. If the father is the "ideal father" Dee wishes for, she can tell him how it is to have these feelings for him. If the father is one who frustrates her, she can then explore her feelings of not getting what she wants from him. The specific path the work takes is typically determined by the clues the member provides or ways in which other members may be triggered by one client's work. Again, we facilitate linking among members so that they can make the fullest use of the group process.

How does this technique benefit Dee? It gives her an opportunity to express feelings that would otherwise be unexpressed. She also gets feedback on the manner in which she presents her thoughts and feelings to her parents and how this manner of presentation may be part of the problem. Other members can learn the importance of how they speak to the significant people in their lives. There are many possibilities for drawing on psychodrama techniques to further Dee's work (see Corey, 2004, chap. 8).

"My father wouldn't talk in English." Carlos has been given the feedback that he sounds abrasive. There is gentleness in his eyes and in the content of his remarks, but he has a way of using his voice that leaves people feeling under attack. He acknowledges the validity of this feedback and wants to explore the theme further.

Drawing on clues from earlier work, the leader can ask Carlos to think how the voice of each of his parents sounded to him when he was a child and to give imitations of each while saying "I'm reluctant to be gentle because _______." The leader may have a hunch that in many ways Carlos is reluctant to be like his father, a kindly man much belittled by Carlos's mother. Sure enough, the imitation of his mother comes across as abrasive. When he starts to present an imitation of his father, Carlos remarks, "My father wouldn't speak in English."

When we are working with bicultural and bilingual clients, we often take the initiative to ask them what language they speak with their family members and friends. Frequently, the techniques we suggest in these cases involve talking in their native language to a significant other (if this person is a key individual in a problem they are exploring). People often display some resistance when asked to work in their native language. Talking in English can distance these clients, whereas their own language may bring back painful associations. Nevertheless, even though the leader does not speak or understand Carlos's native tongue (Spanish), Carlos is willing to proceed by playing the role of his father talking to his mother about what his kindness has cost him. As Carlos proceeds, the leader can be attentive to clues of emotional intensity and urge him to repeat phrases that seem to bring him closer to his feelings. Eventually, Carlos stops after some anger and some crying. By using this technique, the leader demonstrates a willingness to stay with Carlos's emotions even when the content is unknown. The leader can then ask him to review, in English, what his work has taught him. He may say that he is afraid to sound like his father for fear that women will treat him as his father was treated by his mother. He can then try a new voice and say something to each of the women in the group. Other members may comment on how he now seems gentle and yet powerful and attractive. Carlos is not likely to leave the group with a permanent new voice, but he can see the options he has for a different style, and he can acquire considerable insight into how others experience him and the reasons for his abrasiveness.

If other group members have some fluency in the working member's language, we are likely to include them in a role-play exercise. But it is not essential that anyone be familiar with the language. Other members often are deeply touched by this work even though they don't understand the content of what is being said. They are able to pick up the general emotional tone by listening to the member's voice and nonverbal forms of communication.

Once Carlos has finished a piece of his work, ask those members who are emotionally involved to tell Carlos how he affected them. This can be powerful feedback for Carlos and for the members who give the feedback as well. It can also be an ideal place to continue the therapeutic work by inviting others whose own issues are surfacing to talk about themselves. Often all that needs to be said is something like this: "Joyce, you really seem affected by Carlos. Tell him more about what you are feeling." If Joyce says that this work is bringing up painful issues with her father, the leader could say: "Look around the room, Joyce. Who in here do you see that could be most helpful to you right now? How about picking a pair of eyes and talking to that person as your father. Let your 'father' know about some of the pain you've been keeping to yourself." Psychodrama and Gestalt-oriented techniques can be used in this role playing with Joyce (see Corey, 2004, chaps. 8 & 11).

"I feel very burdened." Judy seems tired and weary. At an earlier session she was confronted by Jack for being too quick to reassure him when he was discussing a conflict of his. She revealed then that during her childhood she often took on the role of the family arbitrator, always seeking to smooth over quarrels between her parents. Today, after completing some work with Jennifer involving a great deal of sadness, Judy looks exhausted. When she is asked what is going on with her, she says, "I feel very burdened." To help Judy explore her feelings, the leader may ask her to exaggerate them: "Judy, imagine being weighted down by a heavy chain across your shoulders to which are attached several objects. Allow yourself to feel this weight as you talk and allow it to symbolize how burdened you feel."

The group can be connected to Judy's work by having her stand before each member, one at a time—still feeling the burden of the chain—and complete this sentence: "You burden me by _______." For example, "Jennifer, you burden me by being so sad. I want you to be happy." "Jack, you burden me with your anger. I want everything to be peaceful." After completing this go-around, Judy can make another round using this sentence: "I burden myself by _______." "Jennifer, I burden myself by worrying so much about your being sad." "Jack, I burden myself by thinking I have to be responsible for solving your conflicts." This technique gives Judy some insight into how she is responsible for the way she takes on other people's burdens. (This work with Judy's burdens is very much in tune with the Gestalt approach to groups.)

At one point, standing before Charlene, Judy says "Mother, I burdened myself by wanting you and Dad to get along better." Here the leader can drop the technique in progress and replace it with one designed to pursue the client's lead: "Judy, why don't you just stay there in front of Charlene and continue to talk with her as if she were your mother. Tell her how you burdened yourself as a child."

In work such as that between Judy and her "mother," the leader remains alert to ways to bring other members into the flow of work. It is very possible that the person sitting in for Mother (Charlene) is touched by her own concerns. She may be strongly identifying with Judy. Or she may be very much identifying with the mother and may be resenting what she is hearing from Judy. There may well be other members who are touched by the role play, and it could be most helpful to bring them into the work. If the leader is successful in bringing other members in to do their own work by responding to Judy or Charlene, this may accelerate both women's work. From our perspective, groups are functioning at their best not when we are doing individual therapy with others observing but when we are able to effectively bring in several other people with related themes. Then we are making the best use of the group process as a learning mechanism.

People are often reluctant to give up the things they complain of, and the leader may ask Judy to make a plan of action: "During this coming week, if you find yourself taking on any of the burdens you just relinquished, call one of the members of the group, whoever would be most appropriate, and talk with that person about your struggle." As an adjunct to carrying out this plan, Judy could be asked to spend some time writing in her journal about what she got from this work in the session. This would be a good time to ask Judy what she might come up with by way of additional homework assignments that she could practice during the week. Perhaps she will decide to write an uncensored letter to her mother, which she will not mail, in which she further explores some of the feelings that were tapped in the group session. This strategy keeps the focus of responsibility on Judy for deciding on the ways in which she wants to change and for taking concrete steps to bring these changes about.

The leader in this example draws on several theoretical modalities: Gestalt therapy, in asking Judy to imagine and experience burdens and to bypass resistance by the use of incomplete sentences; the psychoanalytic approach, in focusing on resistance and then insight; and behavior therapy and reality therapy, in asking Judy to make an action plan and giving her homework assignments. The work in this example thus attends to all three areas: thinking, feeling, and doing.

"Here, let me help you." Although not explicitly stated, one member's (Claude's) underlying attitude seems to be "Let me help all of you. I know how you feel, because I was once there myself. I'm sure I can help you." This attitude cuts off exploration. Although it is important for leaders not to find fault with a helping attitude, they need to distinguish between facilitative and nonfacilitative helpfulness. If Claude's behavior is not dealt with, the group will slow down.

To explore Claude's attitude, the leader might say something like this: "Claude, I notice that you seem ready to come to the assistance of people, and yet I very rarely hear you asking for any help for yourself. I remember your saying at the beginning of the group that you were burned out on giving to your family because you got so little in return. It may be that you're behaving in this group in many of the ways you do outside of here. Would you be willing to explore this?" If Claude agrees, the leader can suggest one of these go-arounds (which illustrate Gestalt experiments):

- Go around to each person in the group and say: "The way I could help you is _______."
- If there is somebody in your life who has been a helper, see whether you can become that person, and go around to all members of the group and help them as that person would.
- Pick out someone in the group who in some way reminds you of someone in your family whom you say you are tired of helping. Talk to that person about how it feels for you to help him or her and to get so little in return for yourself.

Why is Claude so anxious about letting others struggle on their own? Does he believe the leader is not taking care of the group's needs and that he has to provide direction? These go-arounds give the leader a chance to discover Claude's motives. Perhaps he has believed all his life that no one will take care of him and that it is his duty to take care of everyone else. He may have been so burdened with taking responsibility for others that he does not see how he can behave any differently. Eventually his work might be directed toward exploring ways in which he would like to be taken care of.

Why ask Claude to exaggerate being helpful when this is the behavior that seems to get in his way? By not trying to talk him out of how he feels, by giving him an opportunity to fully experience how he acts, the leader can get Claude to see clearly the implications of his behavior and to decide whether he wants to continue with his present style.

The leader could also use alternative strategies that involve cognitive restructuring (see Corey, 2004, chap. 13) in working with Claude. For example, the leader might use one of these techniques:

- Ask Claude to list out loud all the reasons he has for helping others. Why is helping others so important? When did he make his decision that his place was to be so helpful?
- Suggest to Claude that he ask for something in return from each person he attempts to help. Here he has an opportunity to experiment with a dimension of his behavior that is undeveloped. This approach calls to his attention his giving style.
- Each time Claude engages in helping behaviors, have group members say to him: "You're helping me again, Claude!" This technique makes use of other members to monitor his behavior.
- Ask Claude to observe his behavior outside the group for a time and record instances in which he puts his own needs in second place. Through this self-monitoring process, he may see ways in which he resists receiving from others.

We are not against a helping attitude, nor would we want to try to get Claude to adopt a "me-first" attitude. Rather, the leader can use these techniques to help Claude discover for himself the restrictive nature of his interactions and how he affects others. Claude's behavior can easily cause resentment in others, for they may feel continually indebted to him while at the same time having little to offer him. Claude may also feel resentment for always having to give.

An intervention that places Claude in the position of the people he is helping may permit him to experience being the "receiver" of support. Claude might gain increased awareness of a part of himself that wants from others what he is giving. Eventually, Claude is likely to recognize that his giving might be blocking others from giving to him. After he gets a clear picture of how his behavior affects others, he can decide whether he wants to change this aspect of his personality. The group provides the context for Claude to see himself as others perceive him, and then he is equipped to decide if and what he wants to change.

"Nobody ever listens to me." Julio says "Nobody ever listened to me when I was a kid, no one ever listened to me in school, no one ever listens to me at home, and I feel that no one listens to me here either." We might begin by asking Julio to pick out some members of the group who he feels are not listening to him and to say what leads him to believe that they aren't listening to him or others. Suppose he gets feedback from the group that suggests he is right—that is, people have found themselves not paying much attention to him when he speaks. We might then try to discover what it is about Julio that causes people not to listen to him. Here are some techniques we might use:

- Ask Julio if there is someone in the group whom he would especially like to have as a listener. He can then talk to that person.
- Ask Julio to go around to each person in the group and complete the sentence "One way I don't listen to myself is _______."
- Ask Julio to become either of his parents and show how he or she might behave in the group.
- If Julio's voice is without much affect, draw this to his attention to see if he can notice his behavior.
- Explore what Julio might gain from not being heard by asking him to work with a sentence starting "If you really heard what I was saying, you would _______."
- Ask some group members to give Julio specific feedback on the ways in which they struggle with him and provide him with some suggestions that would increase his chances of being heard.
- Give him a homework assignment for the next week that will increase his awareness of his underlying beliefs and self-talk.

It might be a mistake to stay too concretely with Julio's first remarks. We want to be ready to pick up clues to what is really bothering him when he says he's not listened to. Maybe he has a history of feeling unloved and unimportant. He may be living out a self-fulfilling prophecy.

By exploring this issue with Julio, we are attempting to (1) get Julio to acknowledge his complaint and give him an opportunity to voice it, (2) get him to exaggerate those aspects of his behavior that might produce the situation of which he complains, (3) have others give feedback that will help him clarify what he might be doing or how others experience him, (4) have him discover where he might have learned to do what he does, (5) give him an opportunity to try out being different, and (6) give him feedback and positive reinforcement for what he chooses to do differently. These techniques are aimed at providing a context for Julio to discover what he does, where he learned it, how his behavior affects others, how he does not listen to others or to himself, and how he could do things differently. (Many of these behavioral techniques and cognitive behavioral techniques are described in more detail in Corey, 2004, chaps. 13 & 14.)

This work may emphasize family dynamics during the client's childhood, but we typically start by looking at present feelings within the group.

Then, if past history becomes relevant, the group members have already been made to feel included in the struggle, and they are ready to stay with the individual's work as he connects his past with his present functioning.

"A part of me wants this, and a part of me wants that." Ambivalence, dichotomies, and polarities are all extremely common in counseling work. Typically, we look for ways in which each part can be expressed and try to assure the client that each part will have a turn to be heard. In this way, the client need not constantly cancel the force of one side by considering the other side simultaneously. Here are some polarities that are often voiced in group work:

- A part of me wants to stay with my family, but a part of me wants to go back to work.
- A part of me wants to push you away, but a part of me wants to have you hold me.
- A part of me loves my Dad, and a part of me hates him.
- A part of me wants to live, but a part of me wants to die.
- Sometimes I feel important; sometimes I feel worthless.
- A part of me trusts you, and yet a part of me doesn't.
- A part of me wants to feel; a part of me wants to go numb.

Polarities can have different meanings. If Fred voices a polarity, are both parts really parts of him, or does he want one thing and introject the point of view of someone else who wants something different? If the two sides seem to genuinely represent him, we would help Fred acknowledge both sides and integrate them. If he clearly wants one side but feels he is supposed to want the other side, our concern is to make this split clear and to present an opportunity for him to reject the foreign side.

One way to clarify the split is to accentuate it. A standard Gestalt technique is to ask Fred to sit in one chair while acting out one side and to sit in a different chair while being the other. This exercise has the advantage of bringing his whole body into play; movement symbolizes doing something rather than being stuck. And using two chairs allows us, and Fred, to clearly identify which side is being expressed. The moment Fred seems to be shifting to the other side in what he says, he should move to the other chair or be asked to do so.

We may look for clues about Fred's preference for one side or the other. Is he comfortable in one chair, tense in the other? We are alert to follow his lead. In using a technique that accentuates polarities, the leader must be aware of when to request that Fred switch sides. The leader may not have to make the request; Fred may be aware of which side he is expressing and change chairs.

Polarities can also indicate that Fred is afraid to make a decision. In this case, however, he may prove to be much clearer about his choice than he wants to acknowledge. Sometimes all we have to say is "Pretend you do know which way to go," "Take a guess," or "What don't you want to know?"

Another approach might be to ask Fred to consciously stay with just one side of his dilemma for the next week and to allow it to become dominant. Or we might ask him to assume that one side wins out and that he must stay with that decision for the rest of his life. How would that feel?

These Gestalt techniques have many possibilities for bringing a struggle involving dichotomies into live action within the group (see Corey, 2004, chap. 11). To include other group members in the work, we might use some of these techniques:

- Encourage others to share dichotomies of theirs that resemble Fred's.
- While Fred is speaking from one side, ask him to select someone else in the group to speak for the other side.
- Divide the group members according to which side of Fred's dilemma they feel closer to, and have a group dialogue.
- Ask Fred to sit in the middle of the group, and let others argue for the various sides.

All of these exercises are aimed at opening up Fred to a deeper exploration of his dynamics. Fred may discover that there is a functional payoff for his being stuck that reinforces his current behavior. Even if Fred never changes, these techniques will help him become more aware of choices that he did not know he had.

"I so much want your approval." People often keep their thoughts to themselves out of fear that if they express themselves they will not gain approval. They struggle with this issue in their everyday lives, and they also bring it to the group. Within a group, if there is a norm about being disclosing, these individuals experience a conflict between the pressure to participate and their desire to withhold for fear that others might not like what they say and do.

Herman has consistently shown a tendency to seek approval indirectly within the group. To explore this issue, the leader asks Herman, "Is there anybody in the group from whom you particularly sense disapproval?" If he thinks that no one in the group disapproves of him, the leader may ask Herman to take on the role of each member of the group, pretend that the person disapproves, and say what disapproving thoughts he supposes this person may have. The rationale for this technique is to uncover his projections. If he picks out someone in the group from whom he senses disapproval, the leader can ask him whom this person reminds him of and then have him speak to the imagined person.

Herman can then pretend that he is that disapproving member and, as such, can say something disapproving to each of the other members of the group. Along with his fear of being disapproved of, Herman may have a strong desire to be critical of others. He may find that his real fear is that others will be as critical as he is. Often those who have an excessive need for approval are also very critical. An expected outcome is that this technique will both open up the group and bring Herman's own dynamics into the open.

"I feel very empty." Adeline says she is afraid to work anymore: "My greatest fear is that if I do look at myself, I'll find that I'm empty and am simply a reflection of what everyone else expects. Now, at least, I can kid myself by saying that maybe I'm not so bad after all; yet if I really looked, I just might find nothing inside. Maybe I don't have anything to offer anyone." In this case, Adeline may feel a void or fear that she is not interesting. She may also be holding back material that she is afraid to acknowledge to herself or the group. In developing a technique for working with her, the leader needs to be prepared to pursue either direction.

It would be a mistake to try to talk Adeline out of what she says she is feeling or to assure her that she does have a great deal going on inside her. Instead, the leader might encourage her to experience even more fully what she feels. To help Adeline express what being empty means to her, the leader can ask her to select a visual image that symbolizes being empty. Suppose she picks a dead tree stump that is hollow inside. The leader can then direct her to become the hollow stump. She may say: "I'm dead and useless. I'm rotten and decaying inside, of no use or value. There's no life left in me, nothing but dead and useless wood." Now the leader can try to have Adeline move from symbolic to concrete language, taking his clues from words she uses that seem to invoke the most feeling in her and from whatever he happens to know already about her: "You mentioned being useless. Would you talk more about ways in which you're feeling useless in your life?" or "You describe yourself as rotten inside. I wonder what's so rotten in there." These promptings may be sufficient to involve her on a feeling level in pursuing these themes. If she does not yet get close to much feeling, the leader can ask her to tell other members something about herself that is rotten, decaying, dead, or empty.

If the leader suspects that what Adeline is saying connects significantly with the concerns of another member of the group, he can ask her to talk to this member about her emptiness. Another possibility is to ask her to talk to a member of the group whom she experiences as being full of life. By doing this exercise, she may discover that she hides behind her sense of deadness because she is jealous of those who seem more alive.

Although people who say they have nothing to offer others often lack confidence, there could be a hidden arrogance in their remark. They may feel that others have nothing to offer them.

As an extension of Adeline's work, she can be asked to write each day for half an hour about all the ways in which she feels empty. She can bring her journal to the next meeting of the group and tell the members how it was to do this assignment and share anything she wants to tell the group. The rationale again is to give her an opportunity to fully experience her sense of emptiness, because once she stops running away from her fear that she is empty, she is more able to determine how much truth there is in it. If she does discover some aspects of her life that are without meaning, she is then in a position to change in ways that could result in a fuller sense of purpose.

Action on Adeline's part is also essential if she expects to change. The leader can challenge her to think of concrete steps she can begin to take to deal with her emptiness in a constructive way. Eventually, Adeline may devise a plan involving new behavior designed to bring some meaning to her life. For example, she may decide to do some things that she has been saying she wants to do but has never made the time to do. Action plans are emphasized by theoretical orientations such as transactional analysis, the behavioral approach, rational emotive behavioral therapy, and reality therapy in groups (see Corey, 2004, chaps. 12–15).

"I feel unappreciated." Bonnie wants to work on her feeling that people do not recognize her or appreciate her. She says: "No matter what I do or how hard I try, I still feel unappreciated. My kids are demanding, and I feel they just use me. What's more, my husband rarely gives me support or tells me that I mean anything to him. He is demanding too, and I'm left feeling that I'm never enough. Even in this group I often feel unrecognized. I feel that I don't count and that what I do in here—or what I am—is not recognized."

We might ask Bonnie to identify and talk to those members of the group (including the leaders) by whom she feels least appreciated. While she is doing this exercise, we pay attention to her style. Is she especially timid or affectless? Is there anything else about her that invites people not to take her seriously? We also want to find out specifically what she means by appreciation and get information about what she may want. We might give her an opportunity to list all the things for which she is not receiving appreciation.

If we suspect from what she says that her feeling of not being appreciated has been with her from childhood, we might ask her to relive a scene when she felt unappreciated. Assume that she focuses on her parents who never appreciated her. She can be herself as a child and talk to her mother and father, using substitutes selected from the group, about what she is feeling: "Go back to that time, be that child, and, as if your parents were here now, say some of the things that you might have wanted to say to them." Bonnie may say: "You don't recognize me for what I do. Nothing I do is good enough for you."

Then we might ask Bonnie to become either of her parents, with someone else in the group playing the part of Bonnie. Bonnie, as one of her parents, can talk about how nothing Bonnie does is good enough. She can imitate her parent's style of talking with her and attempt to express some of the things she fantasizes that her parents may have left unsaid. By having Bonnie's substitute enter into this dialogue, we can involve another person in her work and also give her an opportunity to see how she comes across. The substitute may also give her some ideas for an alternative and potentially more forceful style. This technique encourages her to verbalize some of the feelings she had as a child and then perhaps to discover how she may presently be encouraging people to treat her in the way she felt treated then.

These interventions can be followed with various cognitive approaches aimed at challenging the beliefs that influence Bonnie's behavior. In a number of ways she can be urged to critically evaluate her assumption that regardless of what she accomplishes it will never be enough. This would be emphasized especially in theoretical approaches such as transactional analysis and rational emotive behavioral therapy (see Corey, 2004, chaps. 12 & 14). Some directions for further work can be found in these open-ended questions:

- What will you have to do to feel that you are enough? Who is the person from whom you are seeking this external confirmation, and, even if you attain this validation, will you *then* be enough?
- How are you contributing to your feelings of inadequacy by clinging to the assumption that others must appreciate you?
- How valid is your conviction that you don't count unless others appreciate you?

The goal is to provide a context for Bonnie to think critically about how her assumptions and beliefs determine how she feels. Through the use of cognitive behavioral techniques, Bonnie is likely to feel and behave differently if she successfully challenges some of her self-defeating beliefs.

"I don't like being overweight." Jacob is concerned about being overweight, but at the same time he says he likes who he is and is angry that people consider him heavy: "After all, 50 pounds overweight is not that bad." In this case, the leader needs to attend to the mixed message that Jacob is sending. He says simultaneously that he does not like being overweight and that "50 pounds is not that bad." One approach is to ask Jacob, "If 50 pounds is not that bad, why are you bringing up this concern?" He can be helped to decide what he would like to do with his statement. Does he want to deal with being 50 pounds overweight, or does he want to deal with people who perceive him as being heavy? Might he want to explore both of these topics?

Assume that Jacob would like to deal with both his own concerns about being overweight and people who think he is too heavy. The leader could suggest that he do a go-around and tell each member something that he would like to say to those who tell him that he is too heavy. Once he completes this exercise, there will probably be a number of clues that point the way to another technique aimed at further exploration of how he is affected by those who see him as being overweight.

If Jacob is still willing to pursue his concerns about his weight, it is possible to create an exercise that will assist him in sorting out his feelings and how they affect his self-esteem. The leader can ask him to pick up an object of some weight that is not likely to hurt him and ask: "What would it be like to let go of that weight?" When asked to stand before another member to tell him or her how it is to hold this object, he says: "I can't. I can't move over there easily enough. I'm too inhibited by carrying this heavy thing around."

Eventually, Jacob may pause and reflect on the symbolic significance of the exercise and of his words. The leader can then ask him to repeat some of what he has said, replacing references to the heavy object with references to his own body weight. By speaking symbolically and then concretely, he may be able to reveal the limitations he feels as a result of his weight. When he finally drops the burden he is carrying around, he may remark: "This feels lighter. I can only imagine what it would be like to hold an object weighing

50 pounds. I've become so used to my weight that I had no idea how much of a strain these extra pounds are!"

At the end of the session Jacob may declare his intention to go to a gym, which he was previously embarrassed to do. The leader can ask him to do this homework assignment when in the gym: "Occasionally pick up 50 pounds and reflect on what you learned during your work in the group."

In this example, the resistance Jacob probably would have felt to acknowledging that his extra weight was cumbersome and prevented him from getting close to people was bypassed by being approached symbolically. No one pushed him into losing weight; he had an opportunity to acknowledge his own dissatisfaction with those 50 pounds. It needs to be emphasized that a good deal of trust on the part of Jacob, as well as a high level of trust within the group, are required for this exercise to be effectively and sensitively used.

In our work with members who bring up concerns about being overweight and how it affects their self-image, we typically find that the weight is often symptomatic of a deeper concern. We tend to focus on the deeper struggle, and interestingly, people frequently lose weight when they begin to appreciate themselves for the persons they are. Sometimes members are harshly critical of themselves. If they are able to ease up on their self-critical attitudes and decide for themselves that they want to lose weight, they are more likely to experience success than if they persist with weight-control plans to conform to societal standards of the ideal body.

Props can be used productively to intensify work in other areas as well to help members explore issues that concern them. Here are a few examples:

- Ask a member to hide behind a blanket as he talks about his desire to hide.
- Surround a member with cushions and pillows to emphasize his fear of getting close and his desire for distance.
- Ask participants to collect items that have some personal meaning for them. This object can serve as a reminder for some action.
- Have a member hold a small pillow and talk to it as a child.

All props, of course, are designed for intensifying a member's work, not to entertain the group. At times the participants might be entertained by the use of some props, but this should never be done at a member's expense, nor is this the basic purpose of using props in techniques.

"What I got out of that is _______." Often people quickly forget some of the most significant insights or lessons that emerge in work they do in a group. Some therapists believe people remember what they are ready to remember, but we disagree. Even when catharsis and insight are not followed by a lasting decision to change, clients can profit by thinking about what they have experienced. Tim's emotions are now subsiding, but he has just been through 20 minutes of work on several themes. He began by discussing a conflict he had been having with another member. In the feedback exercise that followed, other members praised him for several of his traits but confronted him for his sarcasm. This feedback led to role playing in which he imitated some of the sarcasm he recalled his mother directing at his father. He then began sobbing over the death of his father, and this work triggered grieving in several members of the group. We ask Tim what he wants to learn from this work. Somewhat to our disappointment he replies: "What I got out of that is that I'm as sarcastic as my mother was and that people don't like me for it." We had hoped he would remember more than just negative feedback, although remembering only negative generalities is a frequent outcome of work in groups. What can we do? Here are some possible techniques we could introduce at this point:

- Ask Tim to review each phase of the work he has just done and summarize the specifics.
- Invite members to tell Tim what they most hope he will remember.
- Ask Tim to take on the role of each person who gave him feedback and repeat, as best he can, what that person said.
- Ask every member who is willing to do so to write in Tim's journal something that he or she wants Tim to remember.
- Ask Tim to describe how he might discount what he got from his work.
- Ask Tim to go around the group explaining to each person who gave him feedback how he might discount that feedback or put it in the most negative light. (For example, he might say he thought June was merely flattering him when she said she found him attractive.)
- Give Tim the homework assignment of writing in his journal about what happened in his work.
- Ask Tim to look around the room and impress on his memory the faces of the members of the group as they look right now after having just been so intensely involved in his work. Ask him to try to recall the way these people look when, in weeks to come, he thinks back on today's work.
- Ask Tim to pretend that his mother and his father are in the room and to role-play each of them in summarizing what has been said.
- Ask Tim to name three or four specific lessons he wants to remember from what he has just experienced and to stand up as he declares these lessons to the group.

In the next chapter we discuss techniques for consolidating lessons learned from a group session and for remembering lessons learned over the whole life of a group. We want to emphasize here that the process of reviewing and consolidating insights and formulating decisions about what to put into practice in daily life should be continually encouraged. The completion of a highly emotional segment of a session is a particularly appropriate time to create and introduce techniques highlighting lessons to be learned.

Concluding Comments

In this chapter we have addressed some themes that a group often explores during the working stage. Our aim is to create and use techniques to facilitate the exploration of material that emerges from the interactions within the group. It is important to take our clues from our clients and then devise techniques that will help them understand how they are thinking, feeling, and behaving. We tend to avoid using planned techniques or structured exercises as catalysts. We hope that we have made the point that techniques are most powerful when they are designed for a specific situation in a group as well as for the personality and therapeutic style of the leader. There is no "right" way to proceed with the material that members produce. Rightness is determined by the ability of the technique to help the group member. There are many useful and creative "right" ways to work with the material members produce. The insight members obtain from a particular technique is more beneficial than an insight gratuitously provided to them by the leader. Throughout this book, we have encouraged creativity and spontaneity in the introduction of techniques. We want to balance that with the hope that leaders will have a rationale and a theoretical underpinning so that a technique is not just a shot in the dark. It is essential that you make it a habit to think about the rationale for the techniques you use and to be in a position to discuss what you hope to accomplish by using them. Finally, at all times techniques must be used with respect and concern for the group participant. Techniques are tools to facilitate self-understanding, not ends in themselves.

Questions and Activities

1. Review our account of the characteristics of the working stage of a group. Think about a group that you have led or in which you have been a member, and describe how it did or did not attain this stage.
2. A member of your group says, "Last week I felt very close to people in the group, and this week I'm feeling as if I want to withdraw." How would you handle this remark? What might you do?
3. Transferences typically occur in most groups. How would you utilize this phenomenon for furthering group work? What kinds of questions could you ask of a member that might elicit the admission of the transference?
4. Explain the connection between how one talks and one's intensity of feeling, and describe some techniques that you think might exemplify this connection. What advantages, if any, do you see in asking a group member to speak in his or her native language? How might you make use of others in the group who share this native tongue? How might you bring into this work others in the room who do not speak that language?
5. Imagine a specific population you might work with, and suppose that a member of such a group were to ask you: "Why do we have to share our feelings? What good does that do?" What would you say? How would your response depend on the population? Would it depend on the stage of the group?
6. In discussing Claude's wanting to be helpful, we proposed that his attitude might have an inhibiting effect on others in the group. Develop a technique designed to explore how others in the group are affected by his style. If you were to ask him to exaggerate being helpful, what

would your theoretical rationale be? What might be the effect of asking him to do an exercise in which he avoids being helpful?

7. People have different ways of expressing their feelings and thoughts, and their styles may work well for them. However, they may be subjected to group pressure to express themselves in other ways. What are your thoughts on this pressure, and what are some responses you might make if you were to observe group pressure to conform to a norm?
8. In the example of Julio, who feels that no one listens to him, we talk about the relevance of past history. If you are using this book as part of a class, have the class divide for a debate on the pros and cons of working on past material in a group. Do you think a behavioral viewpoint excludes considering an individual's past? What about a Gestalt or an existential point of view?
9. When Bettina said she is confused, the leader joined her in her resistance. If you used this technique, how would you explain your rationale to a colleague or fellow student? Invent some techniques for directly confronting resistance and compare these with the approach we suggest.
10. Suppose a member of your group says that you are not sharing enough of yourself. How would you handle this remark if it were made during the working stage of a group? What factors would you take into consideration? To what extent do you see your style as self-disclosing or as stating your own feelings or experiences?
11. Develop a homework assignment for Adeline designed to have her explore her sense of emptiness in everyday life. Develop a different assignment designed to help her challenge any irrational beliefs she may have about her emptiness.
12. During the working stage it is important to continue to ask members to engage in evaluating their progress in the group to determine the degree to which they are attaining their objectives. What are some ways in which you would help members assess their degree of satisfaction with their participation at this stage?
13. We describe Carl as being afraid to get close to people because of childhood injunctions (parental messages). What are some injunctions you received as a child? Are any of your injunctions similar to those of Carl? If so, if you were to self-disclose to him, what might you say? Devise some contracts and homework assignments that you think might encourage him to challenge his injunctions.
14. Assume that Jacob is serious about wanting to lose weight. Do some reading on behavioral approaches to losing weight, and set up a behavioral plan for him. Include devising specific goals, monitoring behavior, and developing reinforcements. How would you assess the effectiveness of your plan?
15. Cheryl says that the real world is not like the group. If you were her group leader and wanted to explain your views on this issue, what would you say?
16. A member shows a reluctance to cry, yet this person seems to be in emotional pain. Do you think it important for him or her to cry? Explain.

17. We are more concerned with what people do not say with respect to fears and feelings than with what they do say in a group. What is your view on this topic?
18. What role would the cultural background of the participants in your group play in deciding which kinds of techniques to use or not to use? Do you have any guidelines for how you might modify certain techniques to fit a group that is made up of culturally diverse clients?
19. Suppose you are leading a group in which several people are simultaneously expressing intense emotion. How might you react to this situation? What might you do if you were frightened by the intensity of their emotions? How would you most like to be as a leader in this context?
20. Do you see the exploration of dreams as valuable in group work? What reservations, if any, do you have about working with an individual's dream in a group? What techniques would maximize the opportunity for others in the group to be involved in working on one person's dream?
21. What kinds of mistakes might you fear making as a group leader? How might your fear get in the way of your trying new techniques? How might you react to mistakes you make in a group?
22. Your group members believe a technique you suggested for one of them was a mistake, but you think your suggestion was appropriate. What would you say or do?
23. We encourage members to gain some cognitive grasp of material they have expressed on an emotional level. We hold that much will be lost if members are not encouraged to think about their work in a group. What is your view, and why?
24. If you have prepared your group during the initial stage, our position is that the group will largely take care of itself during the working stage. Do you agree? Why or why not?
25. What importance do you place on having experienced as a group member any of the techniques that you are likely to introduce in a group that you are leading? To what degree do you think your own experiences as a client in a group can enable you to facilitate a group for others? What are some specific ways in which you can use your membership experience to help members work in depth on their issues?

Guide to Using *Groups in Action: Evolution and Challenges* DVD and Workbook

Here are some suggestions for making use of this chapter along with the working stage segment of *Evolution of a Group*, the first program in *Groups in Action.*

1. *Characteristics of the working stage.* In a concise way, identify the key characteristics of a group in a working stage. During the working stage of the *Evolution* program, how does the group seem different than it did during the initial and transition stages?

2. *Techniques applied to the working stage.* As you view the *Evolution* program, look for specific illustrations of members' work unfolding in that group. See the workbook for a few of the scenarios in the group that are played out during the working stage by various members. What can you learn about the value of role playing, encouraging the group members to work in the here and now, sharing reactions to one another? What is the value of encouraging members to express their feelings over painful issues? What is the value of linking members together with common themes and pursuing work with several members at the same time? How does role playing influence the process of the group? What do you see in the DVD pertaining to how one member's work can be a catalyst that brings others into the interactions? In both the text and the DVD there are examples of symbolically speaking to a parent in one's primary language through role playing. What are you learning about techniques to facilitate self-exploration through symbolically dealing with a parent in a group? How does staying in the here and now enhance the depth of self-exploration?
3. *Working with metaphors.* The DVD demonstrates ways the co-leaders follow a client's lead by paying attention to his or her metaphors. What can you learn about the value of working with metaphors from this piece of work?

Here are some suggestions for making use of this chapter along with *Challenges Facing Group Leaders,* the second program in *Groups in Action.* Below are the themes and vignettes that were enacted in this second segment of the program, *Challenges of Addressing Diversity Issues.*

- What does my culture have to do with my identity?
- I feel different from others in here.
- Sometimes I want to exclude others.
- I struggle with language.
- I resent being stereotyped.
- We are alike and we are different.
- I express myself better in my native language.
- I am colorblind.
- I know little about my culture.
- I want more answers from you leaders.

In *Challenges Facing Group Leaders* the emphasis is on one part of the process of a group that tends to create the most anxiety and concern for group practitioners—the early stages of a group's development. This second program focuses on the challenges at the initial and transition stages. The scenarios that you see in the *Challenges* program can occur at any stage in a group; however, the themes enacted primarily occur during the early phases of a group. If the key tasks of the early stage of a group are not adequately attended to, then the safety in that group is certainly inhibited. In order for a group to achieve the trust necessary to engage in productive work, it is essential that potential problems and concerns of members be identified and addressed—which is the central purpose of this second program.

The second segment of this program is entitled *Challenges of Addressing Diversity Issues.* We address how diversity can affect the group process. Unless members deal with how they perceive their differences, they are not likely to engage in significant personal or interpersonal work. Below are some of the key points that students can be expected to learn about how to work with diversity issues in a group.

- Get the group to talk about how diversity is helping or hindering them in the group.
- The group members learn respect for differences, and they also see areas of commonality.
- It is important for group members to bring up how they feel different from others.
- Leaders need to pay attention to identifying differences and commonalities in the group and the impact of these factors on what is evolving.
- Don't make assumptions about an individual based on his or her cultural background. Always check out your assumptions.
- Don't assume you need to know everything about every member's culture, but remain open to learning what may be salient for each of the members.
- Diversity does not need to be a source of division within a group; rather it can be a unifying factor and can add richness to the group
- Group leaders can never anticipate what will happen. It is never possible to have a perfect lesson plan. What is useful is being present with whatever is happening and not having a preconceived agenda.
- Realize what the group member is saying and its importance to that person. Strive to understand the context in which the member's behavior makes sense.

An exercise for small groups in class. Now that you have viewed the second segment (dealing with diversity), share your observations and reactions. In small groups in class, focus on what you heard and saw, on the interactions that seem to have stood out for you, and the most salient moments of this segment on diversity. What interactions stood out for you? What members were you most noticing and why? What observations did you have about the unfolding of the group process? How is this second segment different from the first segment of this program, if at all? What are you learning about how you might best work with diversity within a group? Pay particular attention to how you are personally affected by the members and the leaders and how that might influence the way you would lead this group. Discuss with one another your reactions to what the co-leaders are doing and what you are learning from this. In your group, share your reactions about what challenges you would expect to face if you were leading this group.

CHAPTER SEVEN

Techniques for the Final Stage

Introduction

In this chapter we discuss termination of individual sessions and of the life of the group, an often-neglected topic. Learning does not happen automatically; it should be fostered and structured throughout the entire life of a group. In an effectively functioning group the members are striving to carry what they are learning in the sessions into their everyday lives. They do this by formulating plans to practice between sessions, by making a commitment to do homework assignments, and by practicing a variety of new behaviors outside of the group.

Perhaps the two most important phases of a group are its beginning and its end: the beginning, because that is where the tone of the group is set; the end, because that is where learning is consolidated and action plans are typically formulated. Leaders pay attention to the endings of every session, yet some specific tasks demand attention as the group approaches its conclusion.

Avoiding acknowledging a group's completion may reflect an unconscious desire on the part of the leader or members not to deal with the role that endings play in their lives. When termination is not dealt with, the group misses an opportunity to explore an area about which many members have profound feelings. Even more important, much of what clients take away from a group is likely to be lost and forgotten if they do not make a sustained effort to review and think through the specifics of work they have done. This is helpful, perhaps essential, to all types of groups, whatever their duration.

In general, the following tasks need to be accomplished during the final stage of the group:

- Members are encouraged to face the inevitable ending of the group and to discuss fully their feelings of separation.
- Members are encouraged to complete any unfinished business they have with other members or the leaders.
- Members are taught how to leave the group and how to carry with them what they have learned and especially how to talk to significant people in their lives.
- Members are assisted in making specific plans for change and in taking concrete steps to put the lessons they have learned into effect in their daily lives.
- Leaders help members discover ways of creating their own support systems after they leave the group.
- Specific plans for follow-up work and evaluation are made.
- Consideration is given to how members might discount a group experience and to teach members relapse prevention strategies.

The more behaviorally oriented models and the action-oriented approaches, such as transactional analysis, behavioral group therapy, rational emotive behavior therapy, and reality therapy (see Corey, 2004, chaps. 12–15), place primary emphasis on these tasks. These theoretical orientations are based on the assumption that group members are responsible for becoming actively involved both in the group and outside of the group sessions. Verbalizations and insight are not enough to produce change. Members need to consolidate their learning, practice homework assignments, and develop a specific action plan if they expect to make significant changes in their lives.

Within the framework of the cognitive behavioral approaches, members are assisted in transferring the changes they have exhibited in the group to their everyday environment. Members are expected to rehearse what they want to say to significant people and to practice alternative behaviors. Feedback from others in the group can be of great value at the final stage in these groups.

Ending a Session

Throughout the life of a group, the leader remains aware of time and teaches the participants how best to use the limited time available to them. Consolidation time is critical at the end of each session. Leaders need to have a sense of timing and not encourage members to bring up new material that cannot be attended to properly toward the end of a given session. Furthermore, leaders need to teach members how to pace themselves so that they do not wait until the end of a session to introduce work that cannot be addressed in the short time remaining.

At times, leaders may open up material when it would be more valuable to start consolidating what has been accomplished. This behavior reinforces the tendency of group members to bring up new material at the last minute (which may be a form of resistance), and it may set a pattern for leaders to extend the sessions. It can also lead members to believe their leader is inadequate or insensitive. For instance, Joan may typically bring up burning issues at the end of the session and then leave complaining of feeling cut off and ignored. In the early stages of a group, these complaints can set the stage for distrust or dissatisfaction.

Asking members to sum up. A good practice is to allow at least 10 minutes at the end of a session, depending on the length of the session and the size of the group, for members to summarize what the session has meant to them individually. Some of these questions may be asked at the end of a session to help members consolidate their learning:

- Could you briefly summarize what this session has meant to you?
- What steps toward your goal are you willing to take between now and our next session to make changes in your life?
- Was there anything unfinished for you today that you would like to continue in our next meeting?
- What was the most important thing you experienced during this meeting?

- Could you summarize the important thoughts or insights you're taking with you?
- What touched you most in other people's work today?
- Before we go, is there any feedback you want to give to someone here?
- What did you learn about yourself?
- Is there anything you thought about working on during this session that you would like to at least mention before we close?
- Did you get what you wanted from this session?
- Are you satisfied with your level of participation in this session?

Questions such as these assist members in identifying specific behaviors they most want to change, both in the group and in daily life, and encourage members to assess what they are doing in the group and their level of satisfaction with the group sessions. It also reinforces members' commitment to make changes.

This practice of making at least a quick check of every member is extremely important, for it challenges members at each meeting to think about what they are both giving to and getting from the group. If they report that they are pleased with what they are experiencing, they can be asked to be specific about what they like and to describe anything they'd like to see more of. If they report that they are not pleased (with the group itself, the leader, or themselves), they can be encouraged to be specific both about what they'd want changed and about their plans for making these changes either in the group or in themselves. If this check is made regularly, members are less likely to be dissatisfied at the termination of the group.

Dealing with unfinished work. What if some work in a session is not going to be finished by the time the group ends? The leader can help bring a sense of closure simply by acknowledging those incomplete explorations or feelings that are left unspoken. Note also that group members often accomplish more than one might suppose in a fairly short period, especially if the leader has been clear about the time constraints. People tend to pace their work to the time they know they have.

If the session has been very emotional, the leader might say something like this: "I know that this has been an emotional session. Before we leave, I'd like each of you to say a sentence or two about what you're leaving with today and where you'd like to take this work during the week and in a future session." Another related approach at this point is simply to ask the client to defer the discussion until the next session. For example, "Since we're running out of time today, would you be willing to reflect on it a bit between now and the next meeting, maybe do some writing, and bring it up again then?"

When a member frequently brings up material toward the end of a session, this pattern needs to be explored. Generally, members will pace themselves fairly well if the leader reminds them occasionally of how much time remains, particularly if the group norm is to keep within the scheduled boundaries. But in spite of one's best efforts, occasionally something will start to develop near the end of a session that will pose a dilemma of either giving up the time structure or seeming to be insensitive. This can often be spotted as it starts to develop, and the leader can defuse the situation somewhat by a comment that makes the problem explicit. For instance: "Alejandro, it seems to me you're getting into some things that we're not going to have time to really explore today. Since we're going to have to stop pretty soon, I wonder if you'd be willing to list the key issues so we can come back to them at the next meeting." Here the leader's phrasing is intended to convey empathy for Alejandro's predicament in being left with the issues coming up; the situation is salvaged about as well as one could hope if the issues are identified and acknowledged and Alejandro is helped to cast things into a form that won't leave him too vulnerable.

It is a mistake to think that unless a concern is brought to a finish that the issue is lost forever. This is rarely the case. If the issue is an important one, it can be returned to, especially if the member makes a commitment to bring it up at the next session when there will be sufficient time to explore it. A leader can remind the client of this commitment at the following meeting by saying: "Alejandro, I remember that during the last session you experienced a lot of intensity related to an issue with your father. I wonder whether you had any more feelings about that or if there is anything you might want to say now to continue with that." The member might say: "I don't feel that anymore." However, if Alejandro is willing to talk for a moment about what he was experiencing during the previous session, without worrying about whether it seems especially here-and-now, he may well be able to get into those feelings again.

In a sense, something is going on at the end of every session. What matters is that whatever is going on be identified and summarized as much as possible. Leaders need to exercise vigilance regarding ending a session. Certain interventions will lead to deeper work, whereas other interventions can help members consolidate what has taken place in a particular session. Regardless of what a leader does, it is unrealistic to think that all members will bring to closure the issues they have raised in a meeting. It is often constructive for clients to leave with a sense of incompleteness, or to have something to think about after the session and to work with in future sessions.

There is a procedure for closing a group session in psychodrama that increases the chances that members will be able to identify and deal with unfinished business. Psychodrama emphasizes allowing enough time for the sharing and discussion phase for each session. Sharing, which comes first, consists of nonjudgmental statements about oneself. Then, after the personal sharing, time is allotted for a discussion of the group process. Members who have engaged in a role-playing enactment are invited to share their reactions to these roles. Others are asked to tell members who participated in a psychodrama enactment how they were personally affected by the work and what they learned from it (see Corey, 2004, chap. 8).

Arranging homework assignments. One technique for closing a session and linking it to the next is to have members announce homework assignments or some means of carrying further the work they have done in a session and then to report on these assignments at the beginning of the next session. Homework can be devised by the members themselves, by the leader, or by other members of the group. In keeping with the spirit of the behavioral approach, it is important for leaders to teach members that the crucial change is the one that takes place in the real world. This is where homework can be helpful. For example, if Maria is fearful of dealing with her professors, she can commit herself to seeking out a professor before the next session and talking with the professor about her fears in the class. If she takes the ultimate responsibility for deciding on the nature of her assignment, she is already taking steps toward change. This example is consistent with the basic tenets of rational emotive behavior therapy, which makes frequent use of activity-oriented homework assignments (see Corey, 2004, chap. 14). These assignments can be given to members by the leader or collaboratively developed through the efforts of the members and the leader. The main point is that insight alone rarely results in behavioral change.

The Adlerian approach to group counseling also places central importance on a reorientation process. From the Adlerian perspective, members are encouraged to take action based on what they have learned in the group. The premise is that insight needs to be translated into action for change to occur. The group becomes an agent in bringing about change because of the improved interpersonal relationships among members. In the Adlerian group, because of the emphasis on equality between members and leaders, homework is likely to be designed in a collaborative manner between the leader and members (see Corey, 2004, chap. 7).

Making your own comments and assessment by the members. Leaders can make a practice of giving their reactions, a group process commentary, and a summary of the meeting toward the end of the session. Leaders might comment on the cohesion of the group, the degree to which members freely brought up topics for work, their willingness to take risks and talk about unsafe topics, the degree to which they interacted with one another (as opposed to speaking only directly to and through the leader), and their willingness to discuss difficult concerns. Leaders might also write notes about each session during the week and then use these comments at the beginning of the next session as a catalyst for linking sessions.

Members can also write down at the end of each session specific topics, questions, concerns, problems, or personal issues that they'd be willing to talk about in the next session. They are thus encouraged to think before the next session about what they've committed themselves to work on. Although some therapists may think that this practice is too forced or planned, it is a way to confront members with their responsibility to use their time.

Another way to close each session is to set aside the last five minutes for members to fill out a brief assessment or rating sheet. This would likely be done on a routine basis in a behaviorally oriented group. These assessments give the leaders a continuing sense of how members are experiencing the group. The rating sheets can be tallied in a few minutes, and the results can be presented at the beginning of the next session, especially if trends are noted. A rating scale from 1 to 10 can be used. Members can rate themselves, other members, and the leaders on some of the following dimensions (the leaders might fill out these forms too):

- To what degree were you involved in this session?
- To what degree did you want to be in the group today?
- To what degree did you see yourself as an active, contributing member of the group today?
- To what degree were you willing to take risks in the group?
- To what degree did you trust other members in the group today?
- To what degree did you trust the group leader today?
- To what degree has today's session stimulated you to think about your problems, your life situation, or possible decisions you might want to make?
- To what degree did today's group affect you emotionally or help you recall emotionally laden events in your life?
- To what degree did you care about other members in this session?
- To what degree were you willing to share what you were feeling and thinking in the session today?
- To what degree did you have clear goals for this session?
- To what degree are you willing to actively practice some new behavior this week?
- At this point, to what degree are you eager to return to the group next week?
- To what degree did you prepare yourself or think about this session before you came today?
- To what degree do you see the group as being alive, goal-directed, and energetic?
- To what degree do you feel safe in this group?
- To what degree are you willing to give others in the group feedback?
- To what degree are you willing to nondefensively take in the feedback you receive and consider it carefully?
- To what degree do you see this group as a positive force in helping you make the changes in your life that you want to make?
- To what degree did you see the group as productive today?

If the leaders add up the results and see clear trends, such as a lack of involvement, a low level of risk taking, an absence of trust, a limited amount of sharing, resistance to returning to the group, and an absence of cohesion, they can open the next session with a remark such as this one: "For the past two weeks most of you have apparently seen this group as a place where you don't feel safe to reveal personal material. Many of you agree that caring is absent, that goals are unclear, and that the energy level of the group is low. I'd like to have us look at this and see what we want to do about it, especially since we have a number of group sessions left." The members can then bring out some of their perceptions and openly evaluate the group, and the members and leaders can make decisions about changing the group's direction. (A more detailed discussion of behavioral assessment is given in Corey, 2004, chap. 13.)

In summary, if we lose sight of the approaching end of a session, we have no choice but to announce, "Well, group, we've run out of time; see you next week." If this practice becomes the norm, we are likely to lose an opportunity to keep the members focused on working toward their goals.

Terminating a Group

It is both ethically and clinically good practice to promote the termination of members from the group in the most efficient period of time. To accomplish this aim, group counselors monitor the progress made by each member and periodically invite the members to explore and reevaluate their experiences in the group.

Preparing for termination. In groups with changing membership, the matter of termination may need to be addressed each week. If Tabita will be leaving the group, her departure needs to be announced ahead of time so that she can deal with her reactions about leaving this group. Also, others in the group will probably have things to say to her about her leaving.

In closed groups with a fixed life span, the issue of termination must be faced well before the last session. Group members should be encouraged to express their thoughts and feelings about the group's ending and to identify what more they want to do before the opportunity is gone. If the group is cohesive, members also need to deal with the sense of loss they may feel when the group is over.

When the end of the group is still some time away, the fact that an end will come can be used to motivate people to work. In the case of a time-limited group, the leaders can point out that the time is passing and that the group will eventually be ending. It is a good practice for leaders to stress the urgency of making full use of the limited time a group has and to help members assess how well they are making use of this time. Members cannot assume that they have plenty of time for getting around to their work. If they do, they will probably feel a sense of dissatisfaction when the final meeting arrives. Some members might say: "It took me a long time to know what I wanted and to feel trusting in here. Now that this group is almost over, I feel I could begin to do some real work."

Leaders can use questions such as these to prompt members to work: "Assume that this is the last chance you're going to have in this group to explore what you want. How do you want to use this time?" or "How do you feel about what you've done, and what would you wish you had done differently?" Here, group leaders can draw upon existential themes such as personal responsibility and the reality of loss and separation as catalysts for encouraging members to evaluate their choices about using the time they have.

In addition, as the end of the group approaches, and preferably not at the last meeting, members can explore feelings they may have about the ending of the group and parallels with separation and loss in their lives. Leaders should not underestimate the likelihood that the group has become for several of the participants a powerful symbol and a focus of hope and change. (A more detailed discussion of other existential concepts that can help members prepare for termination is given in Corey, 2004, chap. 9.)

Leaders also need to be alert to signs that the members are avoiding dealing with the group's ending. When members start introducing topics that they worked on long before, when the work in the group seems lacking in intensity, when there is much lateness, joking, or intellectualizing, members may be signaling through such resistance their unwillingness to leave. The leaders' own willingness to initiate the topic of termination can be excellent modeling here.

Reviewing highlights of the group experience. Much of what members learn in a group will be lost unless some method is used to help them recall these lessons and to apply what they've learned to their everyday lives. One way is to ask members to spontaneously recall moments they shared together: "I'd like each of you to imagine all the events during the time we've been together. Imagine that you have these events on videotape and that you can play back these tapes and actually see and remember what occurred in the group. Now go back and reflect on that first session. What do you remember? How did you experience the group then?" The leader can ask members to share random glimpses of that early session. Then the leader can say: "What were some of the events that you recall most clearly and that had the most meaning for you? Whenever you feel ready, share with the rest of us what you're remembering."

This technique of recalling special moments may bring back to life incidents of conflict in the group, of closeness and warmth, of humor and lightness, of pain, or of tension and anxiety. The more members can verbalize their experiences and the more they can recall what actually happened in the group, the greater their chances of integrating and using the lessons they have learned.

Yallah, for example, says: "I'm thinking about the time when the members here told me that although I appeared tough, they saw a tender side of me. That helped me a great deal to feel that it was acceptable to have feelings, although I must admit that I still have a long way to go before I feel OK about expressing these feelings openly." Sue mentions the time that she confronted the group leader and relates: "I can still feel myself shaking as I got angry at you. That was a new feeling for me, to feel and express my anger to an authority figure, and I learned that the world doesn't fall apart when I show my anger." Samantha recalls: "In one session there was this prolonged silence in the room, which felt terribly uncomfortable to me. I wanted to say something to break the tension in the room. It was important for me to see that the feelings and reactions we were keeping to ourselves were preventing us from going anywhere. I learned that conflict doesn't magically disappear. And I saw that expressing this conflict was all right."

By allowing every member to share significant moments and lessons, this technique helps bring the entire group experience back to all the members. People have a chance to see how their work had an influence on others. The leader can help the conceptualization process by asking members what they learned about themselves and others during these significant moments. This technique of recalling and sharing events is generally a special time and a valuable experience.

Expressing unacknowledged aspects of a group experience. Typically, as a group nears termination, we ask members to clear the air regarding aspects of the group that they might go away viewing negatively. We have concerns about group members who put on a positive front at the end of a group but might later nurse grievances that they never acknowledged. We may express our usual warning that what you don't say may often be more harmful than what you do say. We do not encourage members to say critical things to one another at the very end of a group when there is no opportunity to follow up or work through replies, but we do ask them to be forthright with us, even in the final phase, concerning any features of the group experience they did not find beneficial. Having made every effort to encourage the voicing of honest reactions, we hope that the group members will leave with a generally positive opinion and that they will have stated their gains in ways that will help to make these memorable and lasting.

Techniques for bringing out possible negative reactions that might not be expressed otherwise include asking these questions:

- Suppose it's a year from now and you're sitting around with some friends. The conversation turns to questioning the value of therapy groups. What can you imagine yourself saying?
- Imagine yourself driving home. What might you be thinking about this group?
- As well as reviewing the highlights of this group, we want to take some time to reflect on the moments that were difficult. What were some events that you had doubts about and questioned?
- Is there anything that you have not said that you might regret leaving unsaid?

Exploring the issue of separation. As members terminate an ongoing group, separation becomes a particularly critical issue. As we mentioned earlier, both the member who is terminating and those who are remaining need a chance to express the meaning of what they have shared.

In the case of a closed group, particularly if it has become a cohesive unit, the members often resist leaving. They might be concerned that they will not be as open and trusting with people outside the group. They may wonder whether they will experience the same closeness, caring, nonjudgmental atmosphere, and support once they leave the group. Although leaders cannot deny the importance of recognizing and exploring the feelings of members about separation, they can encourage members to look for support in their relationships outside the group. Leaders might remind members that the closeness they value in the group did not happen by accident. Clients need to recognize what they did to create this special climate. They need to recall that they made a commitment to create an effective group and that they initiated trust. They can then consider how to continue reaching out in similar ways in everyday situations.

Rehearsing new roles. Role-playing techniques can be effective in giving people a chance to practice new behaviors. Of course, the process of rehearsing new roles ought to occur at all the stages of a group, not just during its final phase. Through the technique of rehearsing alternative roles, members can receive feedback from others in the group on the impact they might have, and others can provide alternative behaviors that they may not have thought of. These are examples of behavioral techniques such as behavioral rehearsal, coaching, modeling, and feedback (see Corey, 2004, chap. 13). It should be noted that these techniques are also part of the psychodrama technique of role training (see Corey, 2004, chap. 8).

Some participants want to focus on how they might change others in their lives rather than on what they might change about themselves. Leaders can stress that members have the power to change themselves but cannot directly change others. In the group, for example, Alfonso became aware that he had been holding most of his feelings of both anger and tenderness within himself. He learned that expressing feelings was not unmanly and that terrible consequences didn't follow when he did express himself. Alfonso is concerned for his children, whom he sees as following in his footsteps. Using role playing, Alfonso can practice how he will talk to them. In their feedback the other members remind Alfonso that his children are more likely to begin to express their feelings if he expresses his own emotions to them rather than telling them why they should do so.

Other members feel impatient with their loved ones, wanting them to share the level of awareness they have reached through their group experience. Through the use of role play, they are reminded that their impatience is counterproductive.

Being specific about outcomes and plans. During all group sessions, members should avoid general and global statements and instead be specific and descriptive. During the final stage of a group, being specific is especially important if members are to be clear about what they learned about themselves and how they are going to apply these lessons. If a member says "This group has been very good for me—I've learned a lot and grown a lot," the leader's response might be: "Specifically, what did you learn, and how did you learn this? In what ways has this group been good for you?" If members are specific both about what they have learned and about their plans for change, the likelihood that they will act to change their behavior is increased. Reality therapy offers some very specific guidelines in making and carrying out realistic plans (see Corey, 2004, chap. 15).

Intermember feedback during the final stage also needs to be specific. Members can be discouraged from categorizing others as they give feedback and from saying something they have not said to others before in the group, especially something negative. Introducing new material is not helpful at this time, when the point is to consolidate what has already been seen. A final feedback session is not an opportunity to unload previously unspoken reactions on someone, nor is it a time to shower someone with overly positive generalities. During the final feedback session, what is valuable are specific reactions, impressions, and brief comments. One technique is to ask the people receiving feedback not to respond but to listen carefully to what is being said. Their silence does not imply that they accept the feedback as valid. It simply helps them to hear more clearly than they might if they were to give an immediate response.

Another feedback procedure is to ask members to finish some of the following incomplete statements for each participant:

- My fear for you is _______.
- My hope for you is _______.
- What I'd like for you to remember most is _______.
- One thing I like best about you is _______.
- One thing that brings me closer to you is _______.
- A way I see you as hiding yourself is _______.

Another member can write down the comments for each person receiving feedback and then give the person these notes. Or members can write down their sentence completions in advance of the meeting and then give them to each participant. This procedure makes forgetting these comments less likely.

Projecting the future. The leader can ask members to think of the changes they would most like to have made six months hence, one year hence, and five years hence. Members can then imagine that the entire group is meeting at one of these designated times and can say what they'd most want to say to each other at that time. They can also outline what they will have to do to accomplish these goals.

The technique of future projection is designed to help group members express and clarify concerns they have about the future. However, rather than merely talking about what they would like in a relationship in the future, they can create a future time and place with selected people, bring this event into the present, and get a new perspective on what they want. This intervention, borrowed from psychodrama, focuses members on the changes they would like to make in their lives on both a short- and long-term basis (see Corey, 2004, chap. 8).

Summarizing personal reactions to the group. During the last session of a group, it is valuable for members to make at least brief statements about what it was like for them to be members and to summarize what they are taking with them as a result of the experience. Again, the rationale is that members will carry away more information from a group if they verbalize their reactions and give meaning and perspective to what they've learned. Here are some examples of questions that members might address:

- What has it been like for you to be a member of this group? What has been most helpful (and least helpful) about being in this group?
- What have you learned about yourself? What did you learn about how others view you?
- What were some of the major turning points in this group for you? What were a few of the most significant events for you?
- What are some of the things you most want to say as this group is closing?

This technique allows members to have some idea of what each person is taking away from the group. It also encourages members to think through and to pull together the lessons they have learned. The behavioral and action-oriented theories place primary emphasis on assisting members in identifying what they learned in a group and how they can apply this learning to situations in daily life (see Corey, 2004, chaps. 12–15).

Making contracts. Contracts are useful in helping members identify what, when, and how they want to change a behavior throughout the duration of a group. Some groups are structured around a contract that each member designs. For example, in a typical transactional analysis group the members learn that therapy is a shared responsibility. The members' contracts establish the departure point for group activity (see Corey, 2004, chap. 12).

It is clear that contracts can enable members to state their personal goals in such a way that evaluation of outcomes is possible. Certainly, contracts can be a practical tool for providing direction to members from the beginning of a group, but they also have a place during the final stage of a group. Making contracts to carry out further action once the group ends can be a valuable way to help members try new behaviors in their day-to-day living. The use of contracts is given particular attention in these theoretical orientations to group work: transactional analysis, behavioral approach, rational emotive behavior therapy, and reality therapy (see Corey, 2004, chaps. 12–15). One technique is to ask members to bring a written statement about a change they are willing to make once the group ends. Participants can read their contracts aloud, and others can give specific suggestions for fulfilling the contracts and can comment on the degree to which the contracts seem realistic.

Andres, for example, has come to realize through his group work that he consistently puts himself down with self-defeating remarks and does not try new activities for fear of failure. He knows that he is setting himself up for failure with his internal dialogue. Andres agrees, as part of his contract, to make several signs and tape them to various places in the house. The signs might read: "I will ask for what I want." "I don't have to continue to set myself up for defeat."

Continuing Assessment and Follow-Up

Ethical considerations in evaluation and follow-up. Part of effective practice entails developing strategies to ensure continuing assessment and designing follow-up procedures for a group. Keep these ASGW (1998) "Best Practice Guidelines" in mind when conducting evaluation and follow-up of groups:

> C-1. Group Workers process the workings of the group with themselves, group members, supervisors or other colleagues, as appropriate. Processing may occur both within sessions and before and after each session, at time of termination, and later follow-up, as appropriate.
>
> C-2. Group Workers attend to opportunities to synthesize theory and practice and to incorporate learning outcomes into ongoing groups. Group Workers attend to session dynamics of members and their interactions and also attend to the relationship between session dynamics and leader values, cognition and affect.
>
> C-3. (a) Group Workers evaluate process and outcomes. Results are used for ongoing program planning, improvement and revisions of current group and/or to contribute to professional research literature. Group Workers follow all applicable policies and standards in using group material for research and reports.
>
> C-3. (b) Group Workers conduct follow-up contact with group members, as appropriate, to assess outcomes or when requested by a group member(s).

Conducting follow-up interviews. As a safety check and as a method of assessment, leaders can try to arrange a private interview with each group member a few weeks to a few months after the group ends. Such an interview can be beneficial to the client and can also provide a measure of the group's effectiveness.

The purpose of this session is to determine the degree to which members have met their personal goals and fulfilled their contracts. It's a chance for both leaders and members to discuss the impact of the group, to talk about specific ways of continuing whatever learning was begun, and to discuss any unfinished business or feelings left over from the group. If members are having problems using what they learned, this individual contact is an opportunity to explore ways of dealing with these difficulties. It is also an excellent opportunity for leaders to suggest other groups or individual counseling if it seems appropriate.

Encouraging contact with other members. A technique that can lend support to members as they are practicing new behaviors or completing an action program is to encourage them to periodically contact another member from the group after termination. This contact can be especially important when members find that they have lost their momentum. By calling another member and talking about it, the member gains both support and stimulation. Members can select one or more persons with whom they are willing to

make contact for at least a few months after termination to report progress toward their goals. This is a method of accountability, and a way to establish a support system. Making contact with members outside the group may not be appropriate for all types of groups. Furthermore, it is important that leaders establish with the members that such outside group contact is agreed upon and desired by the members.

Arranging a follow-up session. A follow-up session can take place a couple of months after the end of the group to assess the impact of the group on each of the members. Having such a session is one more way of maximizing the group experience. Because members know that they will meet at some future time to review what they've done, they are more likely to stick to their contracts. We stress in our groups how crucial it is that all members attend the follow-up, regardless of whether they have stuck to their plan for change. Sometimes members who feel that they have let themselves down by not having done what they promised are tempted to "forget" about the follow-up or to claim that they are "too busy." We emphasize that they can learn a great deal from one another by sharing the difficulties they encountered in using what they had learned in the group once they no longer had its support. Leaders can receive important feedback on what members found most helpful.

Suggesting further work. A group experience may be just the beginning for many of the members. Thus, during the final session, the follow-up interview, or the follow-up session, leaders can give a number of suggestions to those participants who wish to continue the work they've begun. These suggestions may include specific recommendations for individual counseling and therapy and recommendations for other closed groups, workshops, or perhaps an ongoing group with some of the same members from the group that just terminated. Leaders can also suggest reading material and perhaps organizations that members can contact for a variety of social activities.

Evaluating a Group

Evaluation form. Leaders can use some type of assessment device to determine the outcomes of a group. We favor devices that tap the subjective reactions of the members both at the final session and at the follow-up session.

There is often a significant difference in how members feel about a group immediately after it ends and how they feel several months later. Feedback in both instances is valuable.

An evaluation form can ask members to assess their degree of satisfaction with the group and the level of investment they had in it; to recall highlights or significant events; to specify actions they took during the group to make desired changes; to specify what techniques were most and least helpful and to suggest changes in the format; and to describe the group after some time has elapsed. Depending on the membership, a structured checklist might be devised, an open-ended letter might be asked for, or a combination of a rating scale and essay questions might be used.

This evaluation procedure is important not only as a way for leaders to measure the effectiveness of the group but also as a way for the members to focus their thinking on what they did during the group and what they received from the experience. Here is one kind of evaluation form that leaders can use to get some idea of the impact of the group on the members.

Member Evaluation Form

1. What general effect has your group experience had on your life?
2. What were the highlights of the group experience for you?
3. What specific things did you become aware of about yourself, your lifestyle, your attitudes, and your relationships with others?
4. What changes have you made in your life that you can attribute at least partially to your group experience?
5. Which of the techniques used by the group leaders had the most impact on you? Which techniques had the least impact?
6. What are some of your perceptions of the group leaders and their styles?
7. What problems did you encounter in the outside world when you tried to carry out some of the decisions you made in the group?
8. What are some of the questions you have asked yourself since the group ended?
9. Did the group experience have any negative effects on you? If so, what were they?
10. Is there anything about groups in general, about this group, or about how it was conducted that you find yourself viewing critically or negatively?
11. How did your participation in the group affect significant people in your life?
12. How might your life be different if you had not been a member of the group?
13. If you had to say in a sentence or two what the group meant to you, how would you respond?

Group leader's journal. Keeping a journal is an excellent idea as it will help you evaluate the progress of the group and assess changes during the stages of its development. Focus not only on what occurs within the group and on the members' behavior but also on your own reactions. Here are some areas that leaders might write about:

- How did you initially view the group? What were your reactions to the group as a whole?

- What were some initial reactions you had to each member? How did any of these reactions or impressions change? What members did you find yourself most wanting to work with? What members did you have difficulty with?
- How was it to lead this group? Did you generally want to be in the group? Did you take your share of responsibility for the group's progress?
- Were there any times that you felt stuck with the group because of a personal concern that you have not explored? Did you find yourself avoiding certain topics because of your own discomfort with these topics?
- What turning points did you see in this group?
- What factors contributed to the success or failure of the group?
- How open were you to taking and considering nondefensively the feedback you received from the members?
- What techniques did you use, and what were the outcomes?
- What were the key events of each session?
- Describe the dynamics of the group and the relationships among members.
- If this group were composed of members very much like yourself, what kind of group do you think it would have been?
- What did you learn about yourself from this group?
- What lessons can you learn from the reactions you had toward specific members?

By keeping such a journal, you can review trends in the group and devise changes in format or techniques for future groups.

You might also type up your observations of each session and give these notes to the members before the following session. Members, too, can be encouraged to keep brief process journals, and you and the members can share your observations. At termination, these journals provide a summary of significant events in the group. In addition, when co-leaders meet to discuss the group's progress, they can refer to their process notes for any differences in perceptions.

Finally, this journal is a good device for generating personal work for you as a leader. You can reserve a section of the journal for writing down whatever comes to mind about unresolved problems in your life. For example, if you become aware of hurt feelings and rejection through the work of some members, you may choose not to work on that problem in the group itself but you can profit from writing in your journal about further work you might do in your own therapy.

Concluding Comments

In this chapter we have emphasized the importance of ending sessions and terminating groups in such a way as to maximize learning and provide an opportunity for growth and change. Reviewing highlights, consolidating lessons, establishing contracts for further work, role playing, getting and giving feedback, and writing are all useful techniques during the final stage.

A group will not promote insight or growth if the leader fails to pay sufficient attention to its ending phases or emphasizes just the experiential dimension of the group process without enlisting the intellects of members to give meaning to what they have experienced.

As a way to review some key points of this book, we suggest that you review the section entitled "In a Nutshell" in Chapter 1. The outline of key ideas and concepts given in that section provides a good review of the material we have addressed throughout all the stages of a group.

We hope that you will find ways to continue learning about groups and practicing leadership skills. The single most important element in becoming a competent group leader is your way of being in a group. If you can be fully present and be authentic, you can be a catalyst for members to engage in introspection, relevant self-disclosure, and risk taking. Your primary function as group facilitators is to support members in their journey of making decisions regarding how they want to live.

As you have seen, techniques are designed as a means to further the agenda presented by the members. Techniques are no better than the person using them and are not useful if they are not sensitively adapted to the particular client and context. The outcome of a technique is affected by the climate of the group and by the relationship between the co-leaders and the members. Techniques are merely tools to amplify emerging material that is present and to encourage exploration of issues that have personal relevance to the members. We encourage you to design techniques that are extensions of yourself. It is our hope that you will continue to use this book as a tool for improving your own ability to create techniques that are suitable for the variety of groups you lead.

Questions and Activities

1. Suppose that your group is almost at the end of a session and several people introduce new and potent material. What might you say or do in response? Can you think of any ways in which you might have set the members up to introduce new material at the end?
2. Describe some techniques or strategies that you might employ to wrap up a particular session of a group.
3. We have said that not acknowledging a group's termination may reflect an unconscious desire on the part of the leaders or members to avoid dealing with separation and endings. How might your own feelings and reactions toward the termination of a group that you are leading affect the manner in which members fully explore their own feelings about the group's termination?
4. What value do you see in homework assignments and other suggestions for action that are designed to give members practice in new behavior outside group sessions? What techniques of this kind might you use in one of your groups?

5. Suppose a member of your group comments on your looking at your watch. What might you say? As a group leader, do you pay attention to time, and do you allow sufficient time at the end of a session for a summary and integration of what has taken place? What are some techniques that you might employ in this regard?
6. When and how might you reintroduce material that a member of your group worked on in a previous session? What are some important considerations here? Would you remind a member of something she seemed to have left unfinished at the prior session? If she indicated that she could no longer get into it, then what would you do?
7. What are some issues you'd want to consider when terminating an open group? a closed group?
8. At the last meeting of a 10-week group, several members urge you to extend the group for a few weeks. What theoretical considerations seem significant to you in this situation? How would you deal with this matter?
9. If you were co-leading a group, what are some of the topics you would want to discuss with your co-leader after the group ends?
10. A supervisor asks you how your group is going. What criteria would you use in replying?
11. We suggest some questions to use on an assessment form for having members evaluate a session. Write an assessment form that would be suitable for a group you might lead. Why would you or wouldn't you use such a form?
12. What are the most important considerations during the final stage of the group? What specific issues would you want members of your group to focus on during this phase, and what techniques could you use to help them do so?
13. A member plans to leave a group that will continue to meet. How do you see this sort of termination as different from the termination of the whole group? What issues are different?
14. Members cannot possibly remember everything they experience in a group. What would you most hope that participants would remember, and what techniques might you use to help them recall and review these lessons?
15. What negative consequences do you think there might be if members do not deal explicitly with the fact that the group is ending? What techniques might you use if you sense participants are inclined to avoid talking about the group's termination?
16. We have said that transfer of learning from the group to everyday life does not happen automatically and that it should be fostered and structured. What are your thoughts on this topic? What techniques would facilitate transferring what was learned in the group to everyday life?
17. Your group is holding a follow-up session several months after its termination. What questions would you most want to ask the participants? What do you see as the significant goals of this meeting?

18. Follow-up sessions may lead participants to feel guilty about progress they have not made. What techniques could you use to enhance the gains that people did make?
19. What are some ways in which you would attempt to evaluate the outcomes of your groups?
20. We discussed the value of group leaders' keeping a journal in which they write process notes as well as describe their personal reactions. What value do you see such a journal having in helping you assess a group's progress? What specific topics do you think you'd most want to include in your process journal? Discuss.

Guide to *Using Groups in Action: Evolution and Challenges* DVD and Workbook

For the *Evolution of a Group* program:

1. *Characteristics of the final stage.* The tasks that need to be accomplished during the final stage of the group are listed on page 164. As you study the ending stage of the *Evolution* program, how do you see these tasks being accomplished in the group?
2. *Techniques for ending a session.* The group in the *Evolution* program provides several illustrations of concluding a day (or a number of sessions) and asking members to think about what they might want to explore in future group sessions. What are your thoughts about how you might end a session? What are you learning about both opening and closing a group session?
3. *Techniques for terminating a group.* Many of the tasks for the final stage addressed in this chapter are illustrated briefly in the *Evolution* group. As you observe the group, ask yourself these questions: How are members in the DVD group prepared for the termination of a group? How do the members conceptualize what they have learned? How does the group seem different at this stage than during the initial phase of its development?

For the *Challenges Facing Group Leaders* program, respond to the following questions:

- If you were leading this group, what kind of specific member behavior would present the greatest challenge to you? Explain.
- If you had to identify what you consider to be the major challenge you expect to face in dealing with diversity within a group, what would this be? Explain.
- From studying this second program, what did you learn that you could generalize to populations you are likely to work with in a group setting?
- What has it been like for you to participate in this second program? What are a few questions that have been raised for you?

SUGGESTED READINGS

Association for Specialists in Group Work. (1998). Best practice guidelines. *Journal for Specialists in Group Work, 23*(3), 237–244. The new guidelines, reprinted in Appendix A, provide a framework for group leaders in planning, performing, and processing a group.

Association for Specialists in Group Work. (1999). Principles for diversity-competent group workers. *Journal for Specialists in Group Work, 24*(1), 7–14. This document spells out areas of beliefs and attitudes, knowledge, and skills and intervention strategies that comprise the dimensions of a diversity-competent group worker.

Association for Specialists in Group Work. (2000). Professional standards for the training of group workers. *Group Worker, 29*(3), 1–10. These training standards identify areas of knowledge and skill competencies required for group workers for task groups, psychoeducational groups, counseling groups, and psychotherapy groups.

Atkinson, D. R. (2004). *Counseling American minorities* (6th ed.). Boston, MA: McGraw-Hill. This edited book has excellent sections dealing with counseling for Native Americans, Asian Americans, African Americans, and Latinos. It helps those who lead groups develop an awareness of cultural issues that affect the members' willingness to take part in group exercises and activities.

Berg, R. C., Landreth, G. L., & Fall, K. A. (1998). *Group counseling: Concepts and procedures* (3rd ed.). Philadelphia, PA: Accelerated Development (Taylor & Francis). This useful book provides practical suggestions on skills required for group facilitation, guidelines for forming a counseling group and facilitation during the early stages, exploration of typical problems in the development of group process, considerations in terminating a group, and groups for various age categories.

Corey, G. (2001). *The art of integrative counseling.* The aim of this book is to present an integrative approach to counseling practice based on working with a client's thinking, feeling, and behaving dimensions. Belmont, CA: Thomson Brooks/Cole.

Corey, G. (2004). *Theory and practice of group counseling* (6th ed.). Belmont, CA: Thomson Brooks/Cole. This text surveys the key concepts and techniques that flow from the major theories of group counseling. It also discusses the stages of groups, group membership, group leadership, and ethical and professional issues in group practice. A student manual with exercises and techniques for small groups is also available.

Corey, G. (2005a). *Case approach to counseling and psychotherapy* (6th ed.). Belmont, CA: Thomson Brooks/Cole. This book presents separate case studies along with ideas for techniques drawn from contemporary counseling approaches. Experts from different orientations demonstrate their styles in working with the same client. The techniques described are also applicable to working with clients in groups.

Corey, G. (2005b). *Integrative counseling*—CD-ROM. Belmont, CA: Thomson Brooks/Cole. This CD-ROM interactive program brings theory into action as it is applied to the case of Ruth. Showing his own integrative style in counseling Ruth, Corey draws on the thinking, feeling, and behaving perspectives, highlighting the value of working with a singular theme from all three modalities of human experience.

Corey, G. (2005c). *Theory and practice of counseling and psychotherapy* (7th ed.). Belmont, CA: Thomson Brooks/Cole. This book describes 11 therapeutic models that are applicable to both individual and group therapy. It also discusses basic issues in counseling, ethical issues, and the counselor as a person. The book is designed to give the reader an overview of the theoretical bases of the practice of counseling. A student manual is available to assist readers in applying the concepts to their personal growth.

Corey, G., & Corey, M. (2006). *I never knew I had a choice* (8th ed.). Belmont, CA: Thomson Brooks/Cole. This book reviews many existential concerns and issues that clients bring to therapy such as those dealing with themes of childhood and adolescence, the struggle toward autonomy, work and leisure, the body and stress management, work, love, sexuality, gender roles, intimacy, loneliness, death, and meaning. The book contains many exercises and activities that leaders can use for their group work.

Corey, G., Corey, M. S., & Callanan, P. J. (2003). *Issues and ethics in the helping professions* (6th ed.). Pacific Grove, CA: Brooks/Cole. A combination of textbook and student manual, this book contains self-inventories, open-ended cases, exercises, and suggested activities. It deals with a range of professional issues pertinent to group work.

Corey, G., Corey, M. S., & Haynes, R. (2003). *Ethics in action: CD-ROM.* Pacific Grove, CA: Brooks/Cole. This self-study program is aimed at exploring ethical decision making, the role of values in the counseling process, and managing boundary issues and multiple relationships. This CD-ROM contains video role-play segments along with exercises for interactive learning and can be used along with either *Becoming a Helper* or *Issues and Ethics in the Helping Professions.*

Corey, G., Corey, M. S. & Haynes, R. (2006). *Groups in action: Evolution and challenges* DVD and workbook. Belmont, CA: Thomson Brooks/Cole. The DVD/workbook package is designed to be used in conjunction with group counseling textbooks. (This interactive self-study program is described in detail in the Preface, and exercises are geared to the video at the end of Chapters 4 through 7.)

Corey, M. S., & Corey, G. (2003). *Becoming a helper* (4th ed.). Pacific Grove, CA: Brooks/Cole. This book deals with the personal and professional lives of helpers. A few of the topics that have special relevance to group counselors include the motivations for becoming helpers, value issues, common concerns facing counselors, managing stress, dealing with professional burnout, and ethical issues in practice.

Corey, M. S., & Corey, G. (2006). *Groups: Process and practice* (7th ed.). Belmont, CA: Thomson Brooks/Cole. Part One deals with the basic issues in group work. In Part Two separate chapters deal with group process issues at each phase in the evolution of a group. Part Three describes specific types of groups for children, adolescents, adults, and the elderly.

DeLucia-Waack, J. L., & Donigian, J. (2004). *The practice of multicultural group work: Visions and perspectives from the field.* Belmont, CA: Thomson Brooks/Cole. This book provides an understanding of multicultural group work from the perspective of group membership and group leadership.

Donigian, J., & Hulse-Killacky, D. (1999). *Critical incidents in group therapy* (2nd ed.). Pacific Grove, CA: Brooks/Cole. The aim of this book is to provide a theoretical rationale that will guide practitioners in working with a variety of groups. The core of the book consists of 12 leading practitioners responding to six critical points in the development of a group.

Earley, J. (2000). *Interactive group therapy: Integrating interpersonal, action-oriented and psychodynamic approaches*. Philadelphia, PA: Brunner/Mazel. This book presents an action-oriented leadership style for group-centered work, with an emphasis on experiential therapy and Gestalt therapy. Some Gestalt therapy concepts explored in this book are awareness and insight, defenses and resistances, presence and contact, and developmental stages of group process.

Feder, B., & Ronall, R. (Eds.). (1994). *Beyond the hot seat: Gestalt approaches to group*. Highland, NY: The Gestalt Journal Press. This book contains some informative articles on the process of Gestalt groups along with techniques to use with various populations. It includes descriptions of art therapy in groups, movement therapy in groups, and marathons.

Gazda, G. M., Ginter, E. J., & Horne, A. M. (2001). *Group counseling and group psychotherapy: Theory and application.* Boston: Allyn & Bacon. This book deals with the foundations of group work, presents an overview of the major theories of group counseling, and describes techniques associated with each of the theories.

Gladding, S. T. (2003). *Group work: A counseling specialty* (4th ed.). Upper Saddle River, NJ: Merrill. This comprehensive book on group work addresses the history of group work, groups for the various age groups, and an overview of the key theoretical perspectives.

Haney, H., & Leibsohn, J. (2001). *Basic counseling responses in groups*. Pacific Grove, CA: Brooks/Cole. The authors structure this group counseling learning system around 15 counselor responses or skills. The package consists of a worktext, a videocassette that illustrates the concepts in the worktext, and a CD-ROM with video segments and Internet links.

Ivey, A. E., Pedersen, P. B., & Ivey, M. B. (2001). *Intentional group counseling: A microskills approach.* Pacific Grove, CA: Brooks/Cole. This text guides readers in a step-by-step process involving specific skills and strategies in group facilitation. A strength of this book is its strong multicultural focus throughout all the chapters.

Jacobs, E. E., Masson, R. L., & Harvill, R. L. (2002). *Group counseling: Strategies and skills* (4th ed.). Pacific Grove, CA: Brooks/Cole. The authors have specific chapters on dealing with problem situations and working with specific populations as well as other general chapters on group process. Several chapters deal with skills such as cutting off and drawing out, making the rounds, and the use of exercises. One chapter is devoted to introducing, conducting, and processing exercises.

Kottler, J. A. (1994). *Advanced group leadership*. Pacific Grove, CA: Brooks/Cole. This book is appropriate for a course that describes how people change in groups and the dimensions of group leadership. Chapters describe group leadership strategies such as risk taking, creative metaphors, the use of humor, and adjunct structures. The final chapter deals with common unethical behaviors in groups.

Kottler, J. A. (2001). *Learning group leadership: An experiential approach.* Boston: Allyn & Bacon. This is a well-written basic text in group facilitation. Some of the chapters include stages of group development, unique leadership skills, when and how to intervene, group techniques and structures, groups for special populations, challenges and obstacles, and group leadership applied to social action.

Leveton, E. (2001). *A clinician's guide to psychodrama* (3rd ed.). New York: Springer. The author offers an excellent view of psychodramatic techniques. Group leaders can benefit greatly from reading the book and following the author's advice for using experimental techniques in group work.

Pedersen, P. (2000). *A handbook for developing multicultural awareness* (3rd ed.). Alexandria, VA: American Counseling Association. The material in this book will be most helpful for group counselors who are interested in expanding their awareness of a multicultural perspective in group work. This useful handbook deals with topics such as becoming aware of our culturally biased assumptions, acquiring knowledge for effective multicultural counseling, and learning skills to deal with cultural diversity.

Shapiro, J. L., Peltz, L. S., & Bernadett-Shapiro, S. (1998). *Brief group treatment: Practical training for therapists and counselors*. Pacific Grove, CA: Brooks/Cole. The focus of this book is on brief, closed groups. The authors describe group process at the preparation, transition, treatment, and termination stages. Individual chapters address the group leader, ethics, group leader training, and co-therapy. In addition, several chapters deal with groups for specific populations.

Smead, R. (1995). *Skills and techniques for group work with children and adolescents*. Champaign, IL: Research Press. This is a very useful handbook for practitioners who work with children and adolescents. The author presents exercises and techniques that can be used in a variety of groups.

Wubbolding, R. E. (2000). *Reality therapy for the 21st century*. Philadelphia, PA: Brunner-Routledge. This is a valuable resource for those interested in learning more about the theory and practice of reality therapy. This book is clearly written, with many practical guidelines for using the principles of reality therapy in practice. It covers a range of techniques that can be applied to group work. The author describes strategies such as creating action plans, the skillful use of questions, and helping clients evaluate their behaviors.

Yalom, I. D. (1983). *Inpatient group psychotherapy*. New York: Basic Books. This is a highly readable book for group therapists who work with both higher- and lower-level inpatient groups. The focus is on general principles of therapy and strategies and techniques of leadership. Techniques are given for a single-session time frame and also for short-term groups with a here-and-now focus.

Yalom, I. D. (1995). *The theory and practice of group psychotherapy* (4th ed.). New York: Basic Books. An excellent and comprehensive text on group therapy, this book presents detailed discussions of the therapeutic factors in groups, the group therapist, issues of transference and transparency, procedures in organizing therapy groups, problem patients, techniques with specialized formats and procedural aids, specialized therapy groups, group therapy compared with the encounter group, and the training of group therapists.

Zinker, J. (1978). *Creative process in Gestalt therapy*. New York: Random House (Vintage). This beautifully written book captures the essence of Gestalt therapy. The author shows how the therapist functions much like an artist in creating experiments that encourage clients to expand their boundaries. This work shows the difference between planned exercises that are imposed on clients and experiments that grow out of the therapeutic process.

APPENDIX A

ASGW "Best Practice Guidelines"

This section presents the Association for Specialists in Group Work (ASGW) "Best Practice Guidelines." These guidelines were prepared by Lynn Rapin and Linda Keel (the co-chairs of the ASGW Ethics Committee) and were approved by the Executive Board on March 29, 1998. The "Best Practice Guidelines" address group workers' responsibilities in planning, performing, and processing group work.

The ASGW is a division of the American Counseling Association, and members are bound to practice within the framework of the *Code of Ethics and Standards of Practice* (as revised in 1995) of the parent organization. The ASGW "Best Practice Guidelines" are meant to clarify and supplement the ACA's *Code of Ethics and Standards of Practice,* not to replace them. The "Best Practice Guidelines" define group workers' responsibilities and scope of practice consistent with current ethical and community standards.

Association for Specialists in Group Work Best Practice Guidelines

SECTION A: BEST PRACTICE IN PLANNING

A.1. Professional Context and Regulatory Requirements

Group Workers actively know, understand and apply the ACA Code of Ethics and Standards of Best Practice, the ASGW Professional Standards for the Training of Group Workers, these ASGW Best Practice Guidelines, the ASGW diversity competencies, the ACA Multicultural Guidelines, relevant state laws, accreditation requirements, relevant National Board for Certified Counselors Codes and Standards, their organization's standards, and insurance requirements impacting the practice of group work.

A.2. Scope of Practice and Conceptual Framework

Group Workers define the scope of practice related to the core and specialization competencies defined in the ASGW Training Standards. Group Workers are aware of personal strengths and weaknesses in leading groups. Group Workers develop and are able to articulate a general conceptual framework to guide practice and a rationale for use of techniques that are to be used. Group Workers limit their practice to those areas for which they meet the training criteria established by the ASGW Training Standards.

A.3. Assessment

a. *Assessment of self.* Group Workers actively assess their knowledge and skills related to the specific group(s) offered. Group Workers assess their values, beliefs and theoretical orientation and how these impact upon the group, particularly when working with a diverse and multicultural population.

b. *Ecological assessment.* Group Workers assess community needs, agency or organization resources, sponsoring organization mission, staff competency, attitudes regarding group work, professional

Source: L. Rapin and L. Keel, "Association for Specialists in Group Work: Best Practice Guidelines," *The Group Worker, 28*(3), Spring 2000, pp. 1–5. [Special insert]

training levels of potential group leaders regarding group work; client attitudes regarding group work, and multicultural and diversity considerations. Group Workers use this information as the basis for making decisions related to their group practice, or to the implementation of groups for which they have supervisory, evaluation, or oversight responsibilities.

A.4. Program Development and Evaluation

a. *Group Workers identify the type(s) of group(s) to be offered and how they relate to community needs.*

b. *Group Workers concisely state in writing the purpose and goals of the group.* Group Workers also identify the role of the group members in influencing or determining the group goals.

c. *Group Workers set fees consistent with the organization's fee schedule, taking into consideration the financial status and locality of prospective group members.*

d. *Group Workers choose techniques and a leadership style appropriate to the type(s) of group(s) being offered.*

e. *Group Workers have an evaluation plan consistent with regulatory, organization and insurance requirements, where appropriate.*

f. *Group Workers take into consideration current professional guidelines when using technology, including but not limited to Internet communication.*

A.5. Resources

Group Workers coordinate resources related to the kind of group(s) and group activities to be provided, such as: adequate funding; the appropriateness and availability of a trained co-leader; space and privacy requirements for the type(s) of group(s) being offered; marketing and recruiting; and appropriate collaboration with other community agencies and organizations.

A.6. Professional Disclosure Statement

Group Workers have a professional disclosure statement which includes information on confidentiality and exceptions to confidentiality, theoretical orientation, information on the nature, purpose(s) and goals of the group, the group services that can be provided, the role and responsibility of group members and leaders, Group Workers; qualifications to conduct the specific group(s), specific licenses, certifications and professional affiliations, and address of licensing/credentialing body.

A.7. Group and Member Preparation

a. *Group Workers screen prospective group members if appropriate to the type of group being offered.* When selection of group members is appropriate, Group Workers identify group members whose needs and goals are compatible with the goals of the group.

b. *Group Workers facilitate informed consent.* Group Workers provide in oral and written form to prospective members (when appropriate to group type): the professional disclosure statement; group purpose and goals; group participation expectations including voluntary and involuntary membership; role expectations of members and leader(s); policies related to entering and exiting the group; policies governing substance use; policies and procedures governing mandated groups (where relevant); documentation requirements; disclosure of information to others; implications of out-of-group contact or involvement among members; procedures for consultation between group leader(s) and group member(s); fees and time parameters; and potential impacts of group participation.

c. *Group Workers obtain the appropriate consent forms for work with minors and other dependent group members.*

d. *Group Workers define confidentiality and its limits (for example, legal and ethical exceptions and expectations; waivers implicit with treatment plans, documentation and insurance usage).* Group Workers have the responsibility to inform all group participants of the need for confidentiality, potential consequences of breaching confidentiality and that legal privilege does not apply to group discussions (unless provided by state statute).

A.8. Professional Development

Group Workers recognize that professional growth is a continuous, ongoing, developmental process throughout their career.

a. *Group Workers remain current and increase knowledge and skill competencies through activities such as continuing education, professional supervision, and participation in personal and professional development activities.*

b. *Group Workers seek consultation and/or supervision regarding ethical concerns that interfere with effective functioning as a group leader.* Supervisors have the responsibility to keep abreast of consultation, group theory, process, and adhere to related ethical guidelines.

c. *Group Workers seek appropriate professional assistance for their own personal problems or conflicts that are likely to impair their professional judgement or work performance.*

d. *Group Workers seek consultation and supervision to ensure appropriate practice whenever working with a group for which all knowledge and skill competencies have not been achieved.*

e. *Group Workers keep abreast of group research and development.*

A.9. Trends and Technological Changes
Group Workers are aware of and responsive to technological changes as they affect society and the profession. These include but are not limited to changes in mental health delivery systems; legislative and insurance industry reforms; shifting population demographics and client needs; and technological advances in Internet and other communication and delivery systems. Group Workers adhere to ethical guidelines related to the use of developing technologies.

SECTION B: BEST PRACTICE IN PERFORMING

B.1. Self Knowledge
Group Workers are aware of and monitor their strengths and weaknesses and the effects these have on group members.

B.2. Group Competencies
Group Workers have a basic knowledge of groups and the principles of group dynamics, and are able to perform the core group competencies, as described in the ASGW Professional Standards for the Training of Group Workers. Additionally, Group Workers have adequate understanding and skill in any group specialty area chosen for practice (psychotherapy, counseling, task, psychoeducation, as described in the ASGW Training Standards).

B.3. Group Plan Adaptation

a. *Group Workers apply and modify knowledge, skills and techniques appropriate to group type and stage, and to the unique needs of various cultural and ethnic groups.*

b. *Group Workers monitor the group's progress toward the group goals and plan.*

c. *Group Workers clearly define and maintain ethical, professional, and social relationship boundaries with group members as appropriate to their role in the organization and the type of group being offered.*

B.4. Therapeutic Conditions and Dynamics
Group Workers understand and are able to implement appropriate models of group development, process observation and therapeutic conditions.

B.5. Meaning
Group Workers assist members in generating meaning from the group experience.

B.6. Collaboration
Group Workers assist members in developing individual goals and respect group members as co-equal partners in the group experience.

B.7. Evaluation
Group Workers include evaluation (both formal and informal) between sessions and at the conclusion of the group.

B.8. Diversity
Group Workers practice with broad sensitivity to client differences including but not limited to ethnic, gender, religious, sexual, psychological maturity, economic class, family history, physical characteristics or limitations, and geographic location. Group Workers continuously seek

information regarding the cultural issues of the diverse population with whom they are working both by interaction with participants and from using outside resources.

B.9. Ethical Surveillance
Group Workers employ an appropriate ethical decision making model in responding to ethical challenges and issues and in determining courses of action and behavior for self and group members. In addition, Group Workers employ applicable standards as promulgated by ACA, ASGW, or other appropriate professional organizations.

SECTION C: BEST PRACTICE IN GROUP PROCESSING

C.1. Processing Schedule
Group Workers process the workings of the group with themselves, group members, supervisors or other colleagues, as appropriate. This may include assessing progress on group and member goals, leader behaviors and techniques, group dynamics and interventions; developing understanding and acceptance of meaning. Processing may occur both within sessions and before and after each session, at time of termination, and later follow up, as appropriate .

C.2. Reflective Practice
Group Workers attend to opportunities to synthesize theory and practice and to incorporate learning outcomes into ongoing groups. Group Workers attend to session dynamics of members and their interactions and also attend to the relationship between session dynamics and leader values, cognition and affect.

C.3. Evaluation and Follow-Up
a. *Group Workers evaluate process and outcomes.* Results are used for ongoing program planning, improvement and revisions of current group and/or to contribute to professional research literature. Group Workers follow all applicable policies and standards in using group material for research and reports.
b. *Group Workers conduct follow-up contact with group members, as appropriate, to assess outcomes or when requested by a group member(s).*

C.4. Consultation and Training with Other Organizations
Group Workers provide consultation and training to organizations in and out of their setting, when appropriate. Group Workers seek out consultation as needed with competent professional persons knowledgeable about group work.

Questions to Consider in Examining the "Best Practice Guidelines"

As you work through these questions, pay particular attention to ways you might apply the "Best Practice Guidelines" to group practice. We hope these questions will raise further questions in your mind and begin the process of developing your own ethical guidelines. Ask yourself what additional guidelines might be included, or consider guidelines you want to challenge. If you were a member of the ASGW Ethics Committee charged with the task of revising these guidelines, which ones would you most want to modify, and why? Do you think the guidelines are complete and comprehensive? Do you see any bias in these guidelines? Do specific areas need to be addressed in more detail for group counselors? Take the time to thoroughly review each of these guidelines in a critical way and discuss the issues raised by them in small groups in class.

1. Scope of Practice and Conceptual Framework
   a. To what extent are you committed to limiting your practice to those areas for which you have met the training criteria established by the ASGW Training Standards?
   b. How well are you able to articulate a general conceptual framework to guide your practice? Can you provide a rationale for the techniques you use?
2. Assessment of Self

a. To what degree are you able to assess your knowledge and skills against those required to effectively lead a specific group?
b. How well are you able to assess your values, beliefs, and theoretical orientation? How do these factors influence your work with groups?
c. To what extent are you aware of your own values, biases, assumptions, and beliefs that most apply to working with culturally different clients?
d. How do you make decisions about which techniques and leadership styles are appropriate to the specific groups you offer?

3. Professional Disclosure Statement
   a. As a group leader, what kind of professional disclosure statement do you believe is appropriate and useful?
   b. What would you most want to include in this document?
4. Group and Member Preparation
   a. What kind of minimal information would you provide to a person wanting to join one of your groups?
   b. How do you think informed consent can best be accomplished in both voluntary and mandatory groups?
   c. What are some legal and ethical issues pertaining to informed consent?
5. Screening Members
   a. Is it unethical to fail to screen?
   b. What are some alternatives when screening is not practical?
   c. How can screening and orientation be handled in mandatory groups?
6. Confidentiality
   a. How would you explain what confidentiality is and its purpose to members of your group?
   b. Under what circumstances are you ethically or legally required to breach confidentiality?
   c. How can confidentiality best be taught to group members and how can it be maintained?
   d. How are you likely to explain to members of your groups that legal privilege does not apply to group work unless it is provided by state statute?
7. Professional Development
   a. What steps might you take to remain current and to increase your knowledge and skill competencies?
   b. As a group worker, when would you seek consultation or supervision?
   c. If you were encountering difficulties leading a group, what steps might you take in getting supervision or consultation?
   d. Can you think of any areas of unresolved personal problems that could impair your professional judgment or inhibit your effectiveness as a group leader?
   e. If you became aware of countertransference issues or personal problems that affected your performance as a group worker, what would you do?
8. Goal Development
   a. What are some ways in which you can help members continually assess the degree to which they are meeting their own goals?
   b. How would you monitor the group's progress toward the group goals and purpose of the group?
9. Diversity
   a. As a group practitioner, what ethical issues might you expect to confront with respect to working with diverse client populations?
   b. To what degree are you willing to seek information regarding the cultural issues of the diverse populations in your groups?
10. Evaluation and Follow-Up
   a. What are some ideas you have for evaluating the process and outcomes of your groups?
   b. Is it unethical to fail to arrange for follow-up meetings?
   c. What are some alternatives to follow-up meetings on either an individual or group basis?

APPENDIX B

Professional Organizations of Interest to Group Workers

It is a good idea to begin your identification with state, regional, and national professional associations while you are a student. Although not all of these organizations have special divisions devoted to group work, they are all at least indirectly relevant to the work of group practitioners. To assist you in learning about student memberships, some of the major national professional organizations are listed here with their contact information and Web sites.

Web Site Resources

American Counseling Association (ACA)
ACA membership provides many benefits, including a subscription to the *Journal of Counseling and Development* and also a monthly newspaper, *Counseling Today*, eligibility for professional liability insurance programs, legal defense services, and professional development through workshops and conventions. Each spring (usually in March or April) ACA holds a national convention. ACA puts out a resource catalog that provides information on the various aspects of the counseling profession, as well as giving detailed information about membership, journals, books, home-study programs, videotapes, audiotapes, and liability insurance. Student memberships are available to both undergraduate and graduate students enrolled at least half time or more at the college level. For further information, contact:

American Counseling Association
5999 Stevenson Avenue
Alexandria, VA 22304-3300
Telephone: (703) 823-9800 or (800) 347-6647 x222
Fax: (703) 823-0252
Web site: www.counseling.org

American Psychological Association (APA)
The APA has a Student Affiliates category rather than student membership. Journals and subscriptions are extra. Membership includes a monthly subscription to a journal, *American Psychologist*, and a newspaper, *APA Monitor*. Each year in mid- or late August the APA holds a national convention. For further information, contact:

American Psychological Association
750 First Street, N. E.
Washington, DC 20002-4242
Telephone: (202) 336-5500 or (800) 374-2721
Fax: (202) 336-5568
Web site: www.apa.org

National Association of Social Workers (NASW)
NASW membership is open to all professional social workers and there is a student membership category. The NASW Press, which produces *Social Work* and the *NASW News* as membership benefits, is a major service in professional development. NASW has a number of informative pamphlets available upon request. For information, contact:

National Association of Social Workers
750 First Street, N. E., Suite 700
Washington, DC 20002-4241
Telephone: (202) 408-8600 or (800) 638-8799
Fax: (202) 336-8311
Web site: www.socialworkers.org

National Organization for Human Service Education (NOHSE)

NOHSE is made up of members from diverse disciplines—mental health, child care, social services, gerontology, recreation, corrections, and developmental disabilities. Membership is open to human service educators, students, fieldwork supervisors, and direct-care professionals. Student membership is $28 per year, which includes a subscription to the newsletter (the *Link*), the yearly journal, *Human Services Education*, and a discount price for the yearly conference (held in October). For further information about membership in the National Organization for Human Service Education, contact:

Chrisanne Christensen
Sul Ross State University
Rt. 3, Box 1200
Eagle Pass, TX 78852
Telephone: (830) 758-5112
Fax: (830) 758-5001
Web site: www.nohse.com

American Association for Marriage and Family Therapy (AAMFT)

The AAMFT has a student membership category. Members receive the *Journal of Marital and Family Therapy*, which is published four times a year, and a subscription to six issues yearly of *Family Therapy News*. For membership applications and further information, contact:

American Association for Marriage and Family Therapy
1133 15th Street, N. W., Suite 300
Washington, DC 20005
Telephone: (202) 452-0109
Fax: (202) 223-2329
Web site: www.aamft.org

Organizations Devoted Specifically to Group Work

Association for Specialists in Group Work (ASGW)

ASGW, a member organization of the American Counseling Association, is one of the most important professional organizations devoted to the promotion of group work. Both regular and student members receive the *Journal for Specialists in Group Work*, which is published in March, May, September, and November; they also receive the ASGW Newsletter, *The Group Worker*, which is published three times a year. The journal and newsletter are excellent sources for staying current in the field of group work. ASGW often holds a national convention in January. For information about joining ASGW, contact ACA:

American Counseling Association
5999 Stevenson Avenue
Alexandria, VA 22304-3300
Telephone: (703) 823-9800 or
(800) 347-6647 x222
Fax: (703) 823-0252
Web site: http://asgw.educ.kent.edu

The ASGW Web page was established to provide a resource base for teachers, students, and practitioners of group work. It includes both organizational information and professional resources (ASGW products, ASGW institutes, and links other Web pages of interest to group workers). *The Professional Standards for the Training of Group Workers* is available on the ASGW Web site.

American Group Psychotherapy Association (AGPA)

AGPA offers both student and regular membership. Membership includes a subscription to an excellent journal, the *International Journal of Group Psychotherapy*, which is published four times a year. The journal contains a variety of articles dealing with both the theory and practice of group therapy. Each year in February the AGPA sponsors a five-day annual meeting that features a variety of institutes, seminars, open sessions, and workshops. For further information about journal subscriptions and membership requirements, contact:

American Group Psychotherapy Association, Inc. (AGPA)
25 East 21st Street, 6th Floor
New York, NY 10010
Telephone: (212) 477-2677
Fax: (212) 979-6627
Web site: www.groupsinc.org

American Society of Group Psychotherapy and Psychodrama (ASGPP)

The American Society for Group Psychotherapy and Psychodrama (ASGPP) is an interdisciplinary society with members from all of the helping fields. The goals of the organization are to establish standards for specialists in group therapy and psychodrama and to support the exploration of new areas of endeavors in research, practice, teaching, and training. The ASGPP holds national and regional conferences, provides a national journal, the *Journal of Group Psychotherapy, Psychodrama and Sociometry*, and offers a number of membership benefits. For further information, contact:

American Society for Group Psychotherapy and Psychodrama
301 N. Harrison Street, Suite 508
Princeton, NJ 08540
Telephone: (609) 452-1339
Fax: (609) 936-1695
Web site: www.asgpp.org

Group Psychology and Group Psychotherapy, Division 49 of APA

Division 49 of the American Psychological Association provides a forum for psychologists interested in research, teaching, and practice in group psychology and group psychotherapy. Current projects include developing national guidelines for doctoral and postdoctoral training in group psychotherapy. The division's quarterly journal, *Group Dynamics: Theory, Research and Practice*, and its newsletter, *The Group Psychologist*, are sent to all members and affiliates. For additional information, contact:

Thomas V. Sayger, Ph.D.
Counseling Psychology, Room 100
Ball Education Building
University of Memphis, TN 38152
Telephone: (901) 678-3418
E-mail: sayger.tom@coe.memphis.edu
Web site: www.pitt.edu/~cslewis/GP2/Hello.html

Codes of Ethics of Professional Organizations

Each of the major mental health professional organizations has its own code of ethics, which can be obtained by contacting the organization. Although ethics codes do not provide answers to ethical dilemmas you will encounter, they do offer general guidance. It is essential that you know the basic content of the codes of your profession and how these apply to you as a group worker.

All of the following codes of ethics and guidelines for practice are available in the booklet, *Codes of Ethics for the Helping Professions* (Brooks/Cole–Thomson Learning, 2003), which is sold at a nominal price when packaged with this textbook:

- ACA Code of Ethics and Standards of Practice
- ACA Ethical Standards for Internet On-Line Counseling
- Ethical Guidelines for Counseling Supervisors
- Code of Ethics of the American Mental Health Counselors Association
- Ethical Standards for School Counselors
- Association for Specialists in Group Work: Best Practice Guidelines
- ASGW Professional Standards for the Training of Group Workers
- ASGW Principles for Diversity-Competent Group Workers
- AAMFT Code of Ethics
- APA Ethical Principles of Psychologists and Code of Conduct
- Ethics of the International Association of Marriage and Family Counselors
- NASW Code of Ethics
- National Board for Certified Counselors, Inc. and Center for Credentialing and Education, Inc.
- Ethical Standards of Human Service Professionals

INDEX